14 September 1990

BEAUTIFUL BY NATURE

BEAUTIFUL BY NATURE

by Li Hillker

Photographs by Marie Hedberg

DAVID & CHARLES
Newton Abbot   London

Beautiful by Nature has been designed and produced by Johnston Co-editions, Gothenburg, Sweden.

World copyright © 1989 Johnston Co-editions, Li Hillker, and Marie Hedberg.

First published in Great Britain by David & Charles 1989

British Library Cataloguing in Publication Data
Hillker, Li   Beautiful by nature
  1. Beauty care. Manuals
  I. Title
  646.7'2

  ISBN 0 7153 9438 X

Reproduction: Repro-Man

Typesetting: concept

Printed in Italy by Graphicom S.r.l., Vicenza,
for David & Charles Publishers plc
Brunel House
Newton Abbot
Devon

CONTENTS

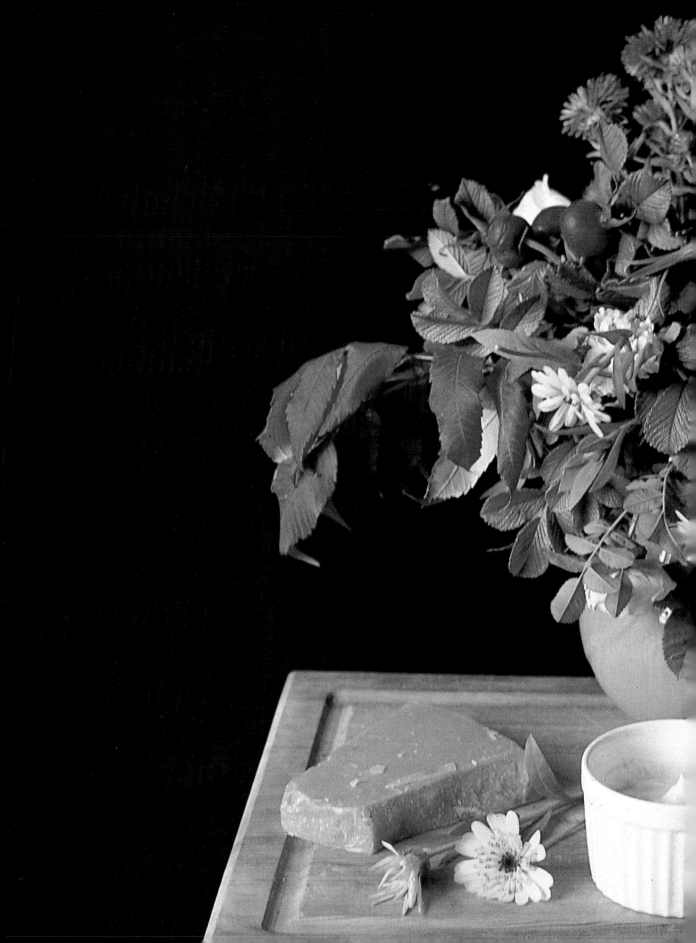

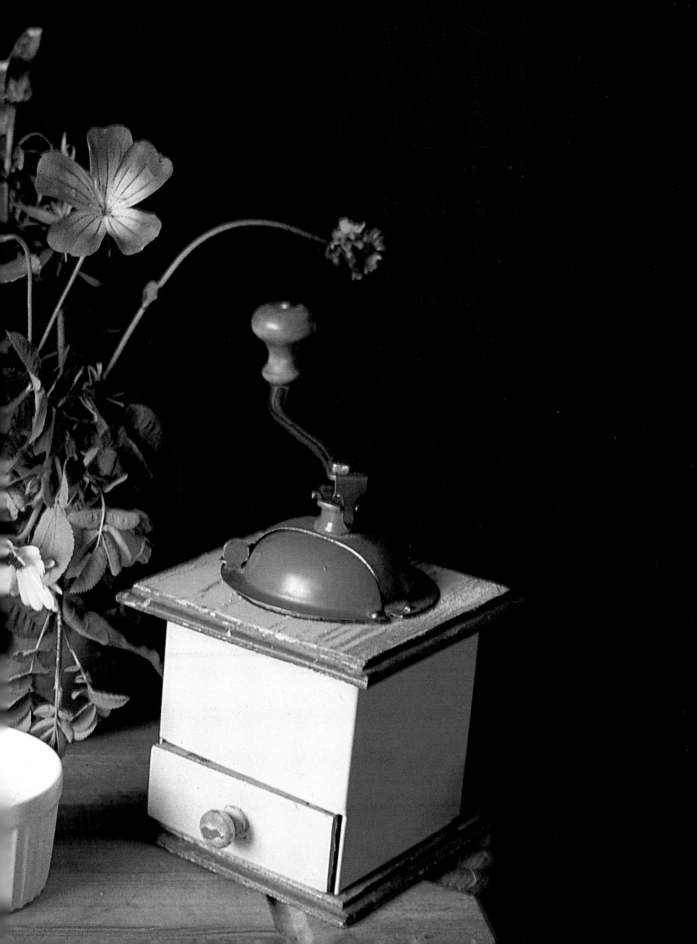

Introduction

Just imagine – a warm morning in early summer, a clear blue sky, and the dew rising like a bridal veil from the trees: a shiver of pleasure runs down one's spine, a feeling of harmony and fulfilment. If only one could feel just like that always, all the year round, no matter what the weather or the time of day!

We all have our little quirks, but the one most of us share is our weakness for make-up of one kind or another. Perhaps it would be more correct to say "still share", for ointments and creams that make us younger and more beautiful have fascinated both men and women all over the world for thousands and thousands of years.

In the early days, it was a question of simple substances, consisting of just one ingredient, or a few at most. As time went by, however, and the art of blending ointments and elixirs of beauty became a respected occupation, the range of skills became broader and broader, and the concoctions became more and more complicated. One of the oldest known recipes was created by the wife of Pharaoh Menes, who lived around 2,900 BC: it is for a cream and a hair dye. The cream, which claimed to keep one's skin young and healthy, contained such things as milk and honey, and the main ingredient for the hair dye was henna.

Inscriptions on ancient graves have revealed that the pharaohs maintained their own cosmeticians, and one of their tasks was to make lipstick for the women. The lipstick had only two ingredients: fat and colouring matter, the latter mainly red. The fat was heated and mixed with the dye, and then the mixture was poured into hollow plant stems and allowed to set.

It is not difficult to see the link with what we now know as lipstick: the main difference is that the manufacture of cosmetics nowadays is a gigantic industry concerned more with chemistry than with craft. Bearing in mind that the industry did not really take off until the twentieth century, however, it is not hard to see that the products made by cosmeticians, chemists, monks or ordinary housewives cannot have been all that bad. Indeed, they must have been pretty effective: for thousands of years now, they have kept women happy and made them feel good.

Whether it is a reaction to the excesses of the chemical industries or the desire for absolute purity, the fact is that there is nowadays a great demand for natural cosmetics. There are not many absolutely natural cosmetics on the market just now: unfortunately, most of them are tainted by chemistry in one way or another. The only sure way is to make one's own cosmetics, and so I hope this book will be of use to people who really want to use nothing but purely natural ingredients in their daily beauty care.

Li Hillker

PART I   BEING PREPARED

All the recipes in this book have been carefully tested, whether they be creams, lotions or face masks. My advice is that when you first start making your own creams and lotions, you should stick strictly to the recipes given; after a while, you will start to get a feel for how the various ingredients react with one another, and then you might find it fun to start experimenting. You'll soon realize the time has come for a few modest improvisations.

Equipment

You should have no difficulty in making your cosmetics at home, in your own kitchen. You will need an electric whisk, and an ovenproof dish holding at least 200 ml (7 fl oz). A stainless steel sieve can be useful: it is just the thing for hanging over the edge of the pan, so that you can suspend your dish in water inside the sieve, rather than standing it on the bottom of the pan. This will prevent water splashing over into your cream and spoiling your results.

It is also a good idea to have a small balloon whisk handy, so that you can continue whisking even when the electric whisk has done its bit; a small set of scales is also useful for weighing the ingredients. Meticulously cleaned, dark-coloured jars and bottles are more or less essential for keeping the products in; any chemist will sell you old medicine bottles at a reasonable price, and they are made to withstand washing in boiling hot water.

In order to achieve the best results with creams, there are a few rules you should always observe:

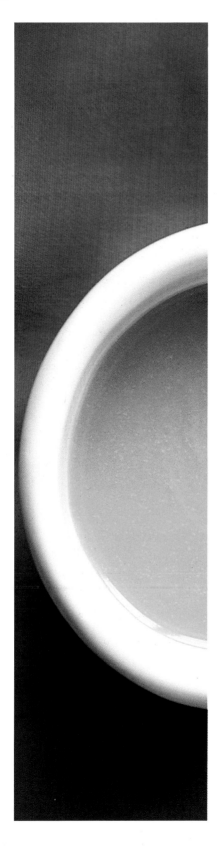

1

Make absolutely certain that all your equipment is properly clean.

2

All the juices you use that are derived from fruit, herbs or vegetables should be carefully boiled and sieved through a fine strainer, in order to eliminate any particles which might conceivably cause the formation of mould.

3

Always use products which have not been subjected to chemical sprays.

4

Any water used should be distilled. Distilled water can be obtained from any chemist.

5

A cream is an emulsion of the "water-in-oil" type – in other words, it consists basically of oil mixed with such things as wax. It is absolutely imperative that the liquid you add to your oil mixture should be at the same temperature – if you add a cold liquid to a hot oil mixture, the emulsification process could well be aborted, and the result could easily be a useless

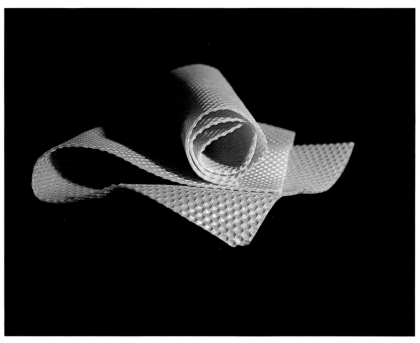

Beeswax is used in many salves and creams.

lumpy mess instead of a nice, smooth cream.

6

Liquid should always be added in stages, a little at a time, stirring vigorously.

7

Always continue whisking the cream until it has cooled down completely, and you are sure it will gel and maintain its consistency. After stirring for

Always whisk your cream until completely cool.

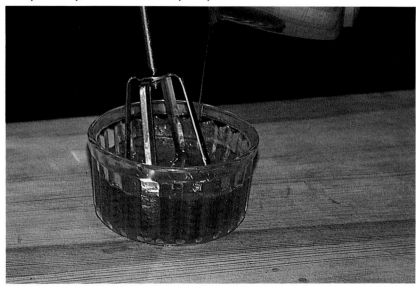

some time with an electric whisk, it is usually sufficient to continue the process with a small balloon whisk.

8

Keep your cream in jars protected from the light and in a cool place, but not in the refrigerator.

9

If you feel you must use preservatives in your creams, I recommend the least harmful of them, sodium benzoate. Sodium benzoate should always be dissolved in the liquid, and not in the oil mixture.

10

Unless you use large amounts of cream, it is a good idea to start by making small amounts: make a little at a time, and use it up. This ensures that it will keep, and obviate the need for preservatives.

11

The ingredients in a cream are sensitive to temperature changes, and so you should be careful to avoid exposing your cream to sudden cooling: this could have an effect on emulsification. What usually happens is that water is precipitated from the oil mixture, and you are left with "two layers" in your jar. It is sometimes possible to re-blend them by whisking, and the process can be helped along by heating.

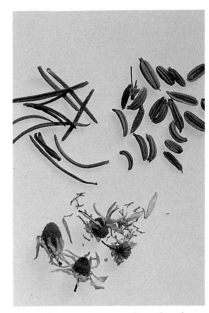

(Above) **Dried rosemary, fennel and camomile. Important natural ingredients in many beauty recipes.**

(Left) **Always start by measuring the ingredients first.**

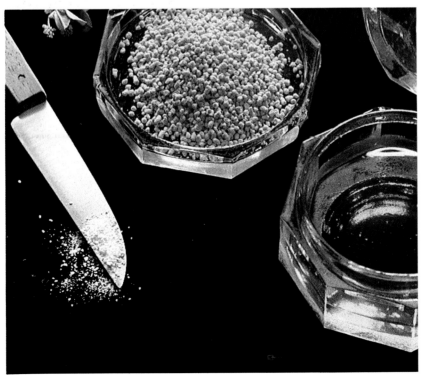

12

The herbs used in a particular recipe may be fresh or dried – indications are given in each individual case. If you decide to use dried herbs rather than fresh ones, however, you should always double the amount given, unless the recipe states otherwise.

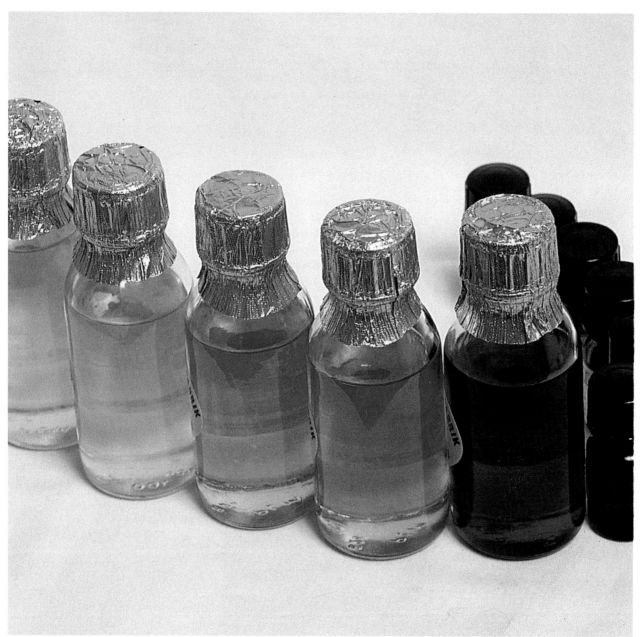

Fragrant oils

Keep your natural fragrant oils cool and dark.

Waxes and oils have a fragrance of their own, and not everyone likes it. The smell of wax can be overcome by adding a few drops of perfume, but this should always be based on natural oils. Do not use synthetic mixtures: they all have a somewhat acrid after-smell which lingers in the senses, unlike the gentle, natural perfumes. Always add the fragrance when your cream, or lotion, is cooling down: heating can alter the perfume, and if you are unlucky, it could become worse.

Measurements
1 tbsp = 15 ml
1 tsp = 5 ml

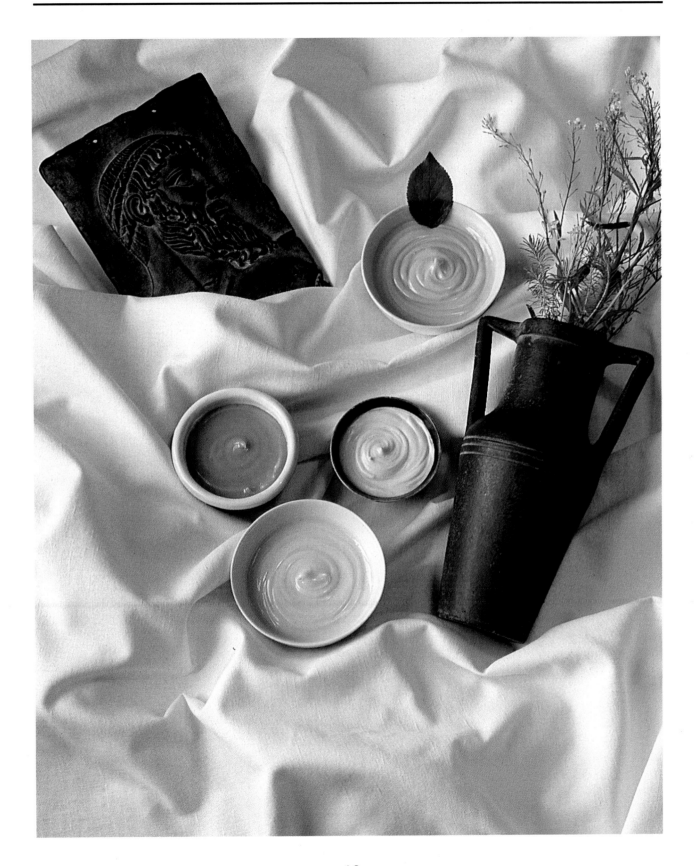

Ingredients, from A to Z

Agar-Agar – a natural solidifying agent made from red algae.

Almond oil – the commonest oil base in both lotions and creams. Mild and healing. Lukewarm almond oil is a good cleanser for delicate baby-skin.

Aloe jelly – a moisture-preserving jelly made from the lilaceous plant Aloe Vera. Aloe jelly has a soothing and healing effect which improves the ability of the skin to absorb oxygen.

Apricot kernel oil – an oil rich in vitamin A, derived from apricot stones. It makes the skin soft and supple.

Avocado oil – used as an oil base in creams and lotions. It is a moisturizer, and is rich in vitamins A, D and E.

Beeswax – taken from the honeycombs built up in the hive by worker bees. Beeswax is an important wax base in creams, but it is not unusual for it to cause allergies: anyone who knows they are allergic to beeswax should replace it in recipes with ordinary white wax.

Borax – a mild substance which kills bacteria, and frequently used as an additive in cosmetics. Borax is a compound based on the element boron (B).

Cocoa butter – occurs naturally in cocoa beans: when cocoa powder is being made, two thirds of the cocoa butter is squeezed out. It is used as a base, or an additive, in the production of creams or lotions. Cocoa butter is a moisturizer.

Coconut butter/oil – the usual oil base in suntan creams. Coconut oil restores fat, and is in fact melted coconut butter.

Fragrant oils – only natural ones should be used in your creams. Start with mild, gentle oils which do not give off too strong a fragrance; a few drops are sufficient for a whole batch of cream.

Glycerol – or glycerine, as it used to be called: a trivalent alcohol which is a colourless and perfumeless viscous liquid used in creams and lotions as a moisturizer. It also improves the consistency of products.

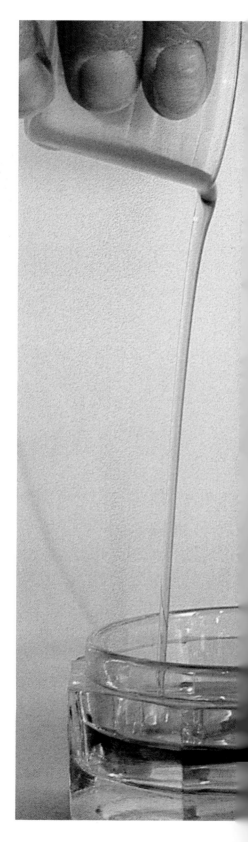

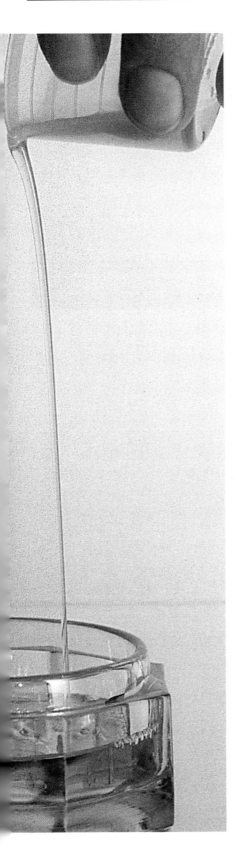

Jojoba oil – one of the more expensive oil bases for creams and lotions. The oil is emollient and is very beneficial for old, wrinkled skin.

Kaolin – a finely ground powder made from soft clay. Kaolin is used primarily in face masks to counter oily skin.

Lanolin – a wool fat with moisturizing and emulsifying properties, which absorbs water easily. Until recently, lanolin was widely used as a base for ointments; it was then discovered that it caused serious allergy problems in women with sensitive skins. Serious manufacturers always state whether their product contains lanolin.

Lecithin – a coarse, fatty powder extracted from soya beans, containing such things as stearic acid, linolic acid and linolenic acid. Lecithin is an excellent emulsifier and hence an important ingredient in lotions which, as distinct from creams, are emulsions of the "oil-in-water" type.

Sesame oil – the usual oil base in sun-tan creams, as the sesame oil naturally filters off the dangerous ultraviolet rays of the sun. Sesame oil is estimated to incorporate approximately protection factor three.

Sodium benzoate – a salt of benzoic acid. Benzoic acid is nowadays made synthetically; it used to be made from benzoic resin, a resin produced by scoring the bark of the benzoin tree. Benzoic resin is yellow and smells of vanilla; when heated, it gives off benzoic acid. Benzoic resin dissolved in spirits is called tincture of benzoin, and was often an ingredient in recipes for ointments in the old days. Benzoic acid and its salt, sodium benzoate, discourages the growth of micro-organisms.

Soya bean oil – a good oil for blending with other oils as it is an effective emulsifier.

Thistle oil – an oil base for creams and lotions, often sold under the name of safflower oil in health food shops.

White wax – a common unctuous base for creams.

All the products named above can be bought at a chemist's or in health-food shops.

No matter how many creams or treatments you apply to your skin, they will have no effect unless the basic cleansing treatment works well. Water is an excellent cosmetic if used in the right way. On its own, lukewarm or cold water moisturizes and soothes, as well as reducing swelling; but it does not remove dirt. Together with soap, however, water cleanses thoroughly; but it is perhaps as well to substitute water and mild cleansing cream occasionally. Alternatively, warm oil can be used – almond oil or groundnut oil. Cleansing oils should only be used at night, however, since particles of dirt lodge very easily in the fat. It goes without saying that cleansing oil should be followed up by "normal" washing the next morning.

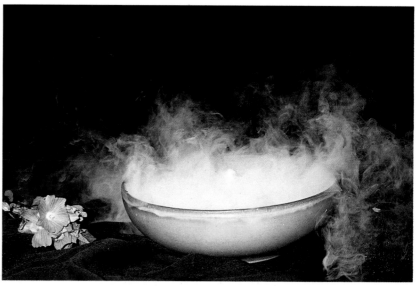

A steam bath refreshes the skin, opening the pores and softening the skin. It is also an important way of bringing much-needed moisture to the skin.

Cleansing before applying a face mask

Face mask treatment has a deep-going effect, which means that it is particularly important for the skin to be thoroughly cleaned before the mask is applied. The most effective way is to use a steam bath, either with water alone, or water and herbs. There is an exception, however: if you have thin blood vessels or extremely superficial skin blemishes, and intend to apply a mask in order to remove them, avoid using a steam bath first: the heat merely aggravates the very things you are trying to cure. After a steam bath, you should not rub or massage the skin, but allow the steam to dry in of its own accord before applying the face mask the moment this is done. If you are going to use a clay mask and your skin is normal or inclined to be on the dry side, it may be as well to avoid using a steam bath and instead to dab away the dirt with a little warm almond oil on a pad of cotton-wool, thereafter applying five layers of a terry towel previously soaked in water as hot as you can bear it. On the other hand, if you have very oily and dirty skin covered in acne, and are going to apply a clay mask, a steam bath in advance can make the treatment more effective.

A simple steam bath

Boil two litres of water and pour it into a wide basin, then place a large towel over your head and lean slightly over the basin. The longer you sit thus, of course, the closer you can come to the basin, since the water is growing cooler all the time. To open the pores completely, you must persist for at least ten minutes, without a break.

Standard steam bath for all types of skin

100 ml (6 tbsp) dried
  camomile
100 ml (6 tbsp) dried mint
1 tbsp fennel seeds
1 tbsp thyme
2 litres (3 1/2 pt) water

Boil the water and pour it over the herbs; it is best to use a stainless steel or heat-resistant basin. Start the steam treatment immediately. An ordinary terry towel draped over the head is easiest, and very convenient to use. Steam the skin protected by the towel for at least ten minutes.

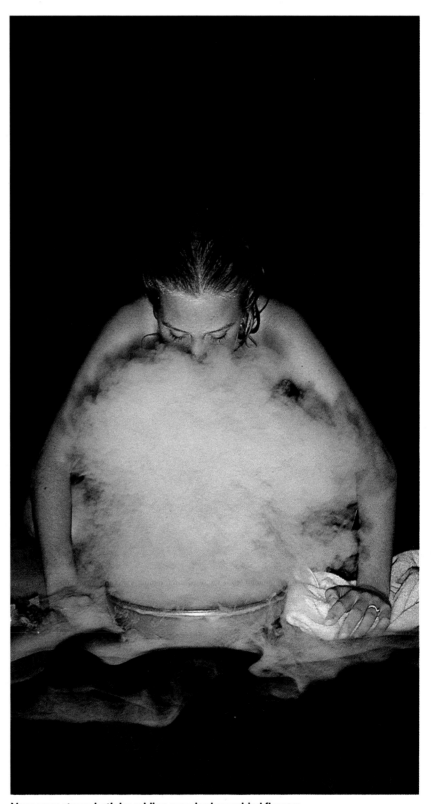

Vary your steam bath by adding new herbs or dried flowers.

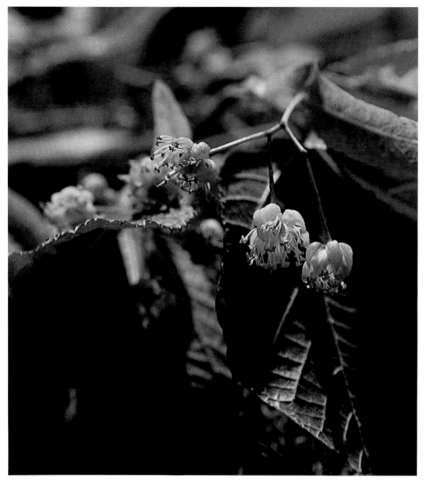

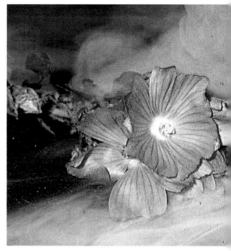

Lime flowers.

Steam bath for tired and jaded skin

100 ml (6 tbsp) dried mint
100 ml (6 tbsp) dried
  camomile
2 litres (3 1/2 pt) water

Proceed exactly as in the previous recipe.

Camomile – a boon for the tired and unfresh complexion.

Steam bath for skin affected by acne

300 ml (1/2 pt) lime flowers
  (fresh)
2 tbsp fennel seed
2 litres (3 1/2 pt) water

Proceed exactly as in the previous recipe.

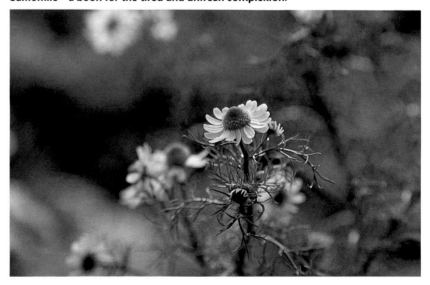

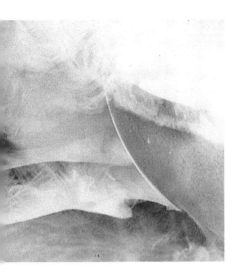

(Left) Always try to use attractive looking accessories and utensils. An aesthetically pleasing atmosphere will help you relax and enjoy your beauty care all the more.

Steam bath for tightening and drying the skin

100 ml (6 tbsp) dried yarrow
100 ml (6 tbsp) mint
2 litres (3 1/2 pt) water

Proceed as above. This steam bath should not be used prior to a clay mask, which itself tightens and slightly dries the skin.

(Below) If you pick your own nettles for use in one of these recipes, be sure to pick only clean nettles. Avoid picking nettles near heavily trafficked roads or industrial areas.

Healing steam bath

200 ml (7 fl oz) dried
     comfrey (leaves)
3 tbsp dried fennel seed
2 litres (3 1/2 pt) water

Proceed as above.

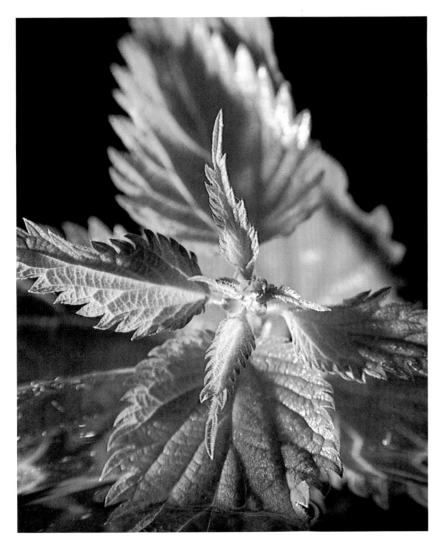

Deep-cleansing steam bath

3 tbsp dried fennel seed
200 ml (7 fl oz) dried nettles
2 litres (3 1/2 pt) boiling
     water

Proceed as above.

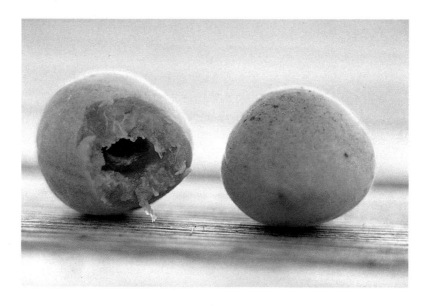

Softening, smoothing and filled with fruit: apricots have everything your skin needs.

— PART II THE RECIPES

Banana

Lemon

Orange

Peach

Apricot

Papaya

Strawberry

Rosehip

Cocoa

Coconut

Almond

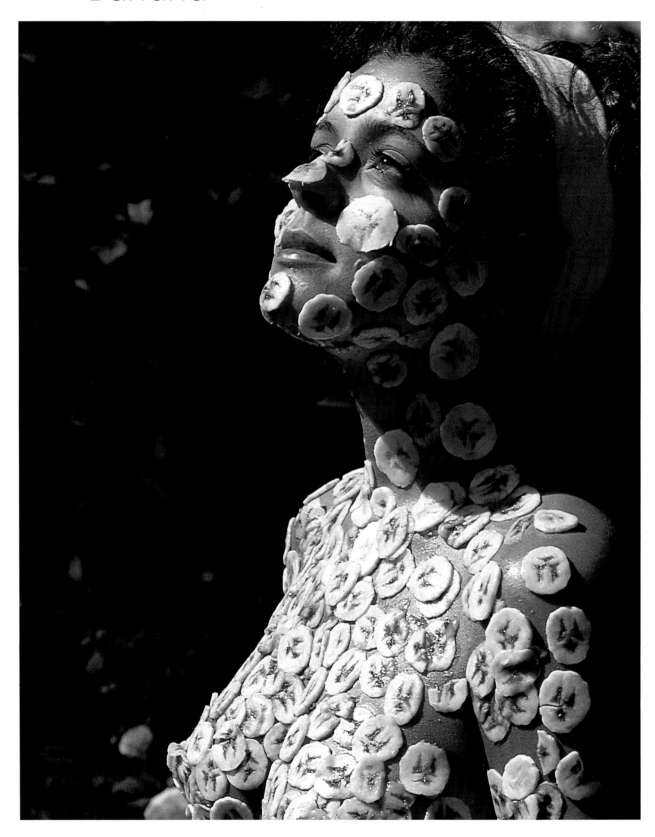

Bananas are a splendid skin-softener, besides having a moisturizing effect and being very nourishing for the complexion. Bananas are most effectively and simply used in face masks.

Skin that has been too much in the sun needs moisture, and the most simple and natural way imaginable – thin slices of banana – is also one of the most effective.

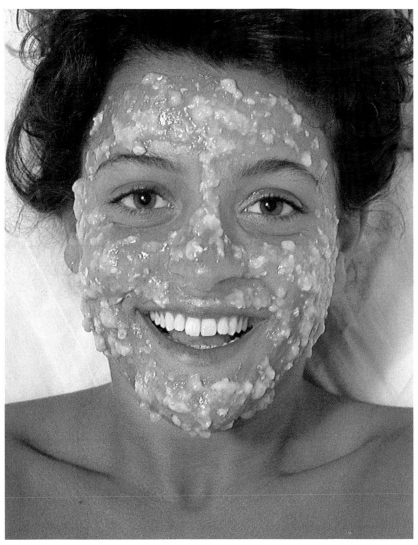

This banana mask moisturizes the skin while giving it a light scrub.

Banana mask

1 banana
1 tbsp honey
5 tbsp oatmeal
distilled water (optional)

Beat the banana to a pulp, then add the honey and the ground oatmeal. Mix the ingredients to form a smooth paste, adding a little distilled water if the mask becomes too hard. Apply the face mask to moist skin, and leave in place for at least fifteen minutes. Rinse with luke-warm water.

Variations

Finely ground sweet almonds can be used instead of oatmeal, and glycerol can replace the honey. If your complexion is greasy and you require a gentle tightening effect, use yoghurt instead of both the honey and the water. Another variation is simply to apply slices of banana directly onto the skin: this smoothes and softens a complexion slightly dried by the sun.

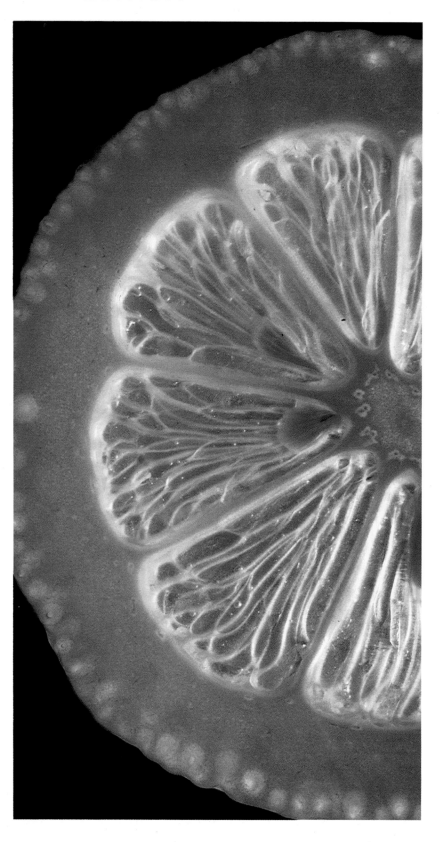

Lemon has both a smoothing and an invigorating effect on the skin. Sore nipples bathed in lemon are soon healed. Lemons are also excellent for oily skin, and cure chapped patches on such places as elbows and knees.

Pulverized, well-brushed lemon peel makes an effective deodorant.

An excellent hand lotion can be obtained by mixing 1 part fresh lemon juice with 5 parts glycerol.

Excessively oily parts of the face can be normalized by using a little segment of lemon. Rub carefully, then rinse with lukewarm water.

Astringent mask

2 tbsp kaolin powder
1 tbsp yoghurt
3 tbsp lemon juice

This face mask is only recommended for people with very greasy skin.

Mix all the ingredients and apply the face mask immediately, avoiding the area around the eyelids. Leave the mask in place for about ten minutes, then rinse with lukewarm water.

Cleansing lemon mask

3 tbsp lemon juice
2 tbsp almond oil
200 ml (7 fl oz) oatmeal
distilled water

This lemon mask cleanses and contracts the pores. The oatmeal introduces a gentle abrasive effect into the treatment, which is good for skin plagued by grease and acne.

Mix the ingredients and add water to form a smooth paste. The oatmeal is made either by grinding rolled oats in a mixer, or simply by rubbing the oats between one's hands for a while. Apply the face mask, and let it remain in place for about fifteen minutes, then rinse with lukewarm water.

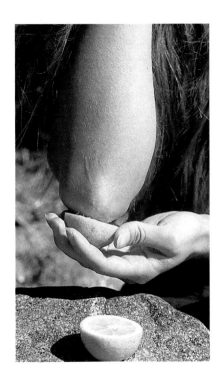

Lemon cream

30 g (1 oz) white wax
1 tbsp almond oil
50 ml (3 tbsp) coconut oil
2 tbsp glycerol
125 ml (7 1/2 tbsp) lemon
  juice
3 tbsp distilled water
1 tsp borax
1 pinch sodium benzoate, if
  desired

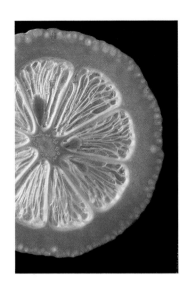

This is a cleansing cream which helps tighten the pores, mainly for people with oily skin.

Melt the wax into the oils by means of a water-bath, then stir gently with a balloon whisk until the mixture is clear and the wax has melted completely. Mix the lemon juice and the distilled water in a saucepan, add the borax, and heat the liquid until it reaches roughly the same temperature as the oils. If a preservative is required, it should also be dissolved into the liquid – not into the oil mixture. Add the glycerol to the oil mixture, then remove the dish from the water-bath. Add the lemon liquid very slowly, whisking thoroughly all the while with an electric whisk, and continue whisking until it is clear the cream has stabilized, that is, until it holds together and no longer "glides apart". At this point, you may replace the electric whisk with a small balloon whisk, and continue beating until the cream is thoroughly cool. Use a spoon to transfer it into properly cleaned jars, and keep in a cool place.

Orange

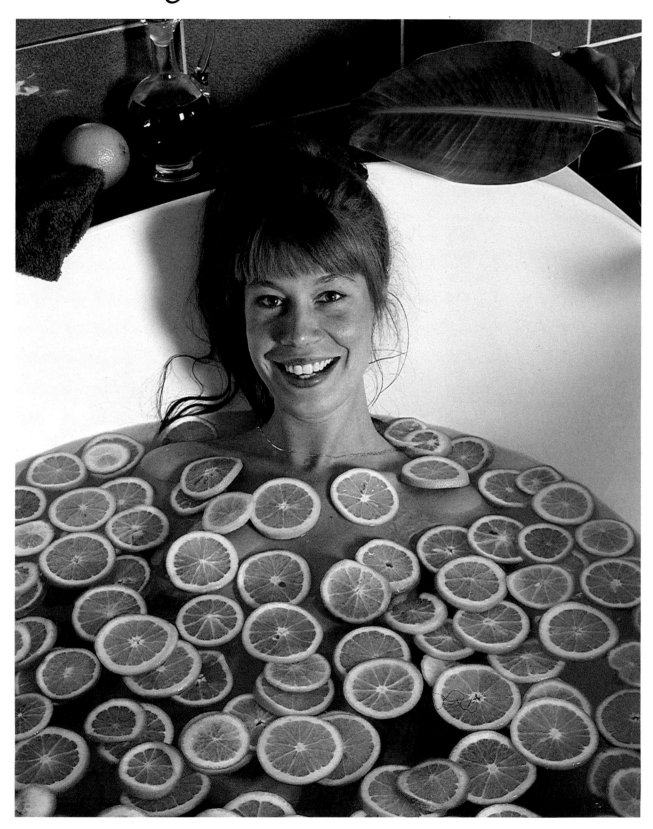

Oranges liven up tired skin, and the high vitamin C content has a soothing effect. Oranges also keep the skin supple. Orange-blossom water is often used in lotions and creams, but since it is hard to find sufficient quantities of orange blossom for one to make one's own orange-blossom water, an acceptable sub-stitute has to be found: a mixture of genuine orange-blossom oil and water will suffice. Real orange-blossom water can in fact be found in especially good health-food shops, herbal chemists, and shops specializing in natural cosmetics: it is always worth shopping around.

Orange mask

1/2 orange
2 tbsp glycerol
3/4 tbsp sweet almonds
2 tbsp cream

This has a smoothing and softening effect, and is very good for dry skin. It can also be applied to the neck.

Peel and liquidize the orange. Mix it with finely ground sweet almonds. Whip the cream gently and blend with the glycerol. Whisk vigorously for a short while. Apply the mask, and leave for twenty minutes. Rinse with lukewarm water: do not rub, but rinse liberally.

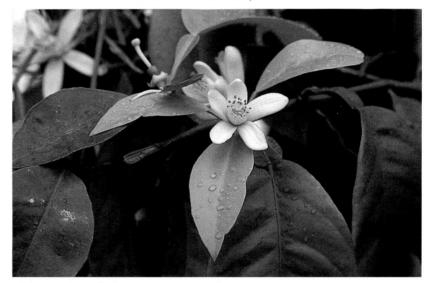

Orange-blossom water

1 litre (1 3/4 pt) distilled water
1 tbsp orange-blossom oil
1/4 tsp borax

Orange-blossom water can be used all over the body. It is good for dry complexions, as an enlivening agent in face masks, and it soothes badly sunburnt and chapped skin. Orange-blossom water can also be used in creams and lotions.

Heat up the water and add the oil drop by drop, then whisk until the mixture has cooled somewhat. Use a spoon to add the borax, and pour the water into meticu-lously cleaned bottles. Keep in a cool, dark place.

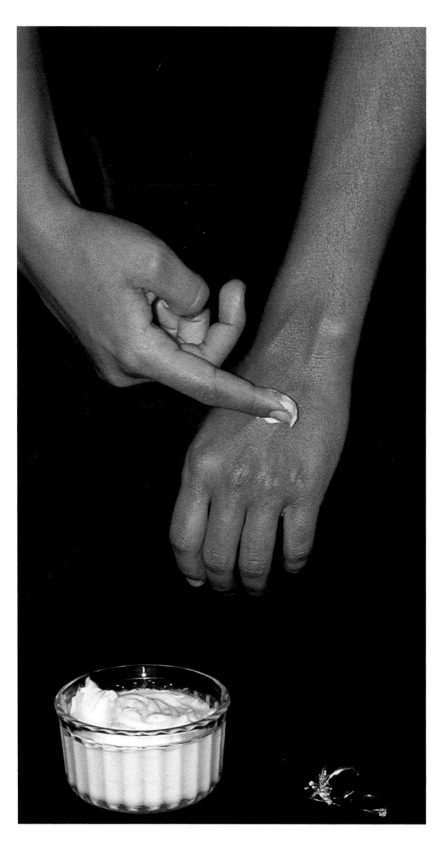

Orange hand cream

5 g (1/2 tsp) white wax
3 tbsp thistle oil
2 tbsp coconut oil
1 tbsp lanolin
2 tbsp glycerol
100 ml (6 tbsp) orange-
  blossom water
1 teaspoon borax
1 pinch sodium benzoate,
  if desired

Melt the wax, oils and lanolin in a water-bath. Whisk with a balloon whisk. Heat the orange-blossom water but do not boil: if a preservative (sodium benzoate) is required, dissolve it in the orange-blossom water. Use a spoon to add the borax to the orange-blossom water, and keep it warm until the oil mixture is homogeneous. Both the wax and the lanolin should have dissolved completely. Add the glycerol to the oil mixture, and stir gently. Remove it from the water-bath, and add the orange-blossom water a little at a time. Whisk with an electric whisk until the cream has stabilized and cooled down altogether. Spoon the cream into dark-coloured, thoroughly cleaned jars, and keep in a cool, dry place.

Peach

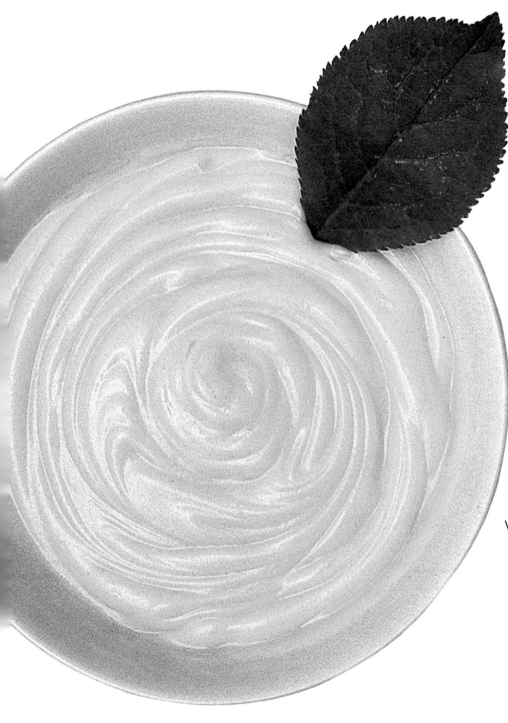

The juice of peaches refreshes tired and jaded skin. Peach has a marked moisturizing effect, and also helps to heal the skin. Dry skin becomes responsive and elastic if treated regularly with peach juice.

Peach cream

10 g (1 tsp) white wax or
    beeswax
2 tbsp almond oil
3 tbsp wheatgerm oil
1 tbsp glycerol
6 tbsp pure pressed peach
    juice
1/2 tsp borax
1 pinch sodium benzoate,
    if desired

Peach cream is especially good for dry and ageing skin, but can of course be used by people with any kind of skin. It is an exceptionally good moisturizer.

Melt the wax and oils together in a water-bath, stirring gently with a balloon whisk until the mixture is smooth and clear. Meanwhile, heat the peach juice (for comments on pressing, see page 35), and dissolve in it the borax and also the preservative, if desired. Then add the glycerol to the oil mixture, stirring all the time. Keep on stirring for a while, then remove the dish from the water-bath and add the hot peach juice a very little at a time. Whisk vigorously with an electric whisk while doing so, and when all the juice has been added, keep using the electric whisk until the cream has almost cooled down altogether. You may now replace the electric whisk with a small balloon whisk until the cream is cold. At this point, a few drops of fragrant oil may be added.

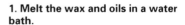
1. Melt the wax and oils in a water bath.

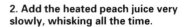
2. Add the heated peach juice very slowly, whisking all the time.

3. Add the wax/oil mixture, while whisking vigorously.

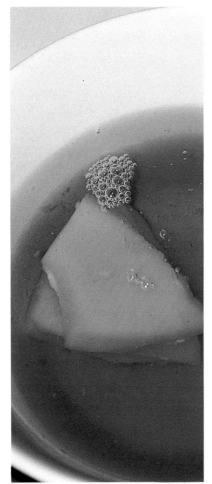

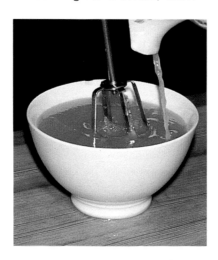

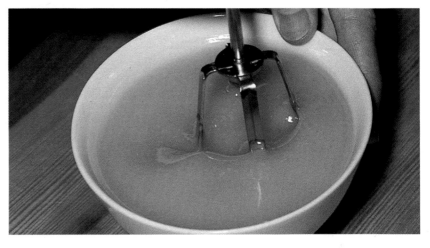

Peach mask 1

1 peach
2 tbsp thistle oil
1 tbsp granulated lecithin
1 tsp honey
50 ml (3 tbsp) distilled
    water
arrowroot flour or finely
    ground sweet almonds

This peach mask is a super-moisturizer, thanks in no small measure to the lecithin, which can if necessary be replaced by egg-white.

Peel and pulp the peach – a mixer is ideal for this purpose. Heat the oil and the granulated lecithin in a water-bath, stirring gently until all the granules have dissolved. Then mix the honey, the peach pulp and the distilled water, add the oil mixture, and whisk vigorously – an electric whisk is not necessary. Introduce as much arrowroot flour or finely ground sweet almonds as necessary in order to produce an easily workable paste. Apply the face mask and leave in place for about half an hour before rinsing off with lukewarm water.

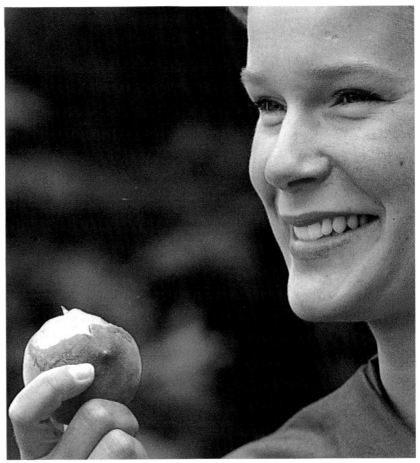

Peaches help the skin to retain its natural moisture.

Peach mask 2

2 peaches
50 ml (3 tbsp) thick cream
1 tbsp kelp
oatmeal, if required

A toning, softening and thoroughly refreshing face mask. Those with oily skin would be well advised to substitute yoghurt for the cream.

Press out the juice from the peaches: better results are obtained by using an electric juice press than doing the job by hand (see section on papaya mask). Mix the cream and the kelp with the peach juice, and add a little oatmeal if you want a firmer mask. Apply the mask, and leave in place for about thirty minutes before rinsing away with lukewarm water.

Apricot

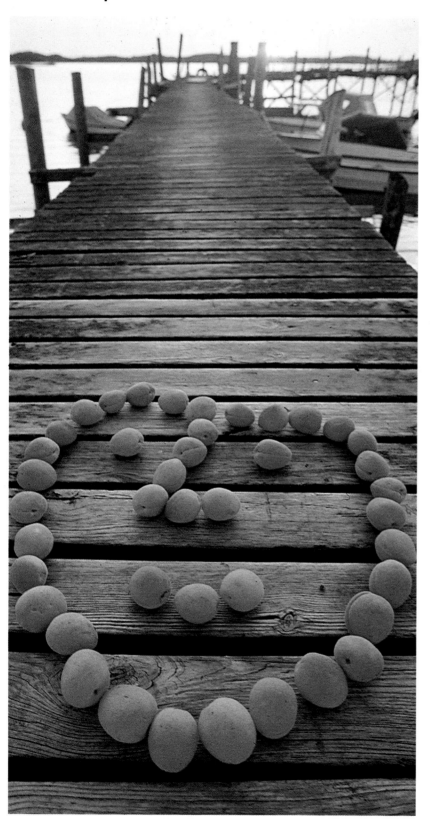

Apricots are rich in vitamin A and therefore have a healing effect on the skin. Apricot kernel oil is used in creams and face masks: it is an excellent cleanser and restores life to dry skin.

Apricot cream

10 g (1 tsp) beeswax
4 tbsp apricot kernel oil
2 tbsp coconut oil
2 tbsp glycerol
3 tbsp distilled water
1 pinch sodium benzoate, if desired

This cream is softening, suits all types of skin, especially dry skin, and its smoothing effect means it can be recommended for ageing skin.

Melt the beeswax and the oils in a water-bath, stirring gently all the time with a small balloon whisk until the mixture is smooth and clear. Add the glycerol. Meanwhile, heat the distilled water, but do not boil. If a preservative is desired, it should be dissolved in the hot water. Remove the oil mixture from the water-bath and add the hot water extremely slowly. Whisk with an electric whisk until the cream is homogeneous and has cooled completely; a balloon whisk is probably sufficient. Spoon the cream into a thoroughly cleaned dark-coloured glass jar, and keep in a cool, dark place.

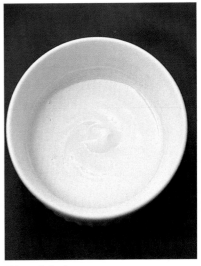

(Above) **Apricot cream.**

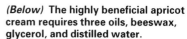

(Below) **The highly beneficial apricot cream requires three oils, beeswax, glycerol, and distilled water.**

Apricot mask

4 apricots (dried)
3 tbsp yoghurt
distilled water (optional)

An apricot mask is nourishing and invigorating for the complexion. It is also an excellent after-sun mask, since it removes sunburn.

Let the apricots lie in the open for twenty-four hours, then reduce them to a fine mousse together with the yoghurt – a mixer is perfect for this purpose, if one is available. Add the distilled water if desired, but the consistency should not be "runny". Apply the apricot mask and leave it in place for about twenty minutes, then rinse with lukewarm water.

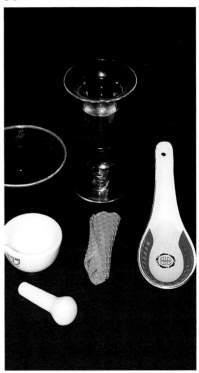

Papaya

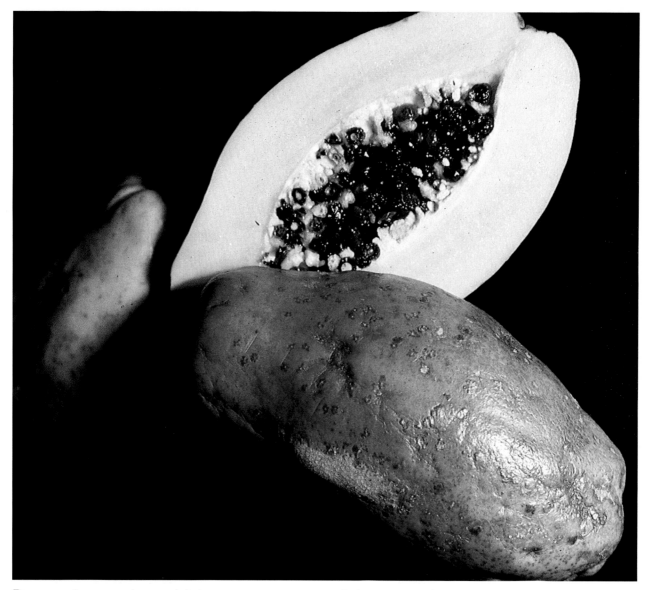

Papaya is a melon which grows on trees. It is grown in most tropical countries, and is imported into other countries most of the year round. It is rich in vitamins A and C. Papaya juice is used for bleaching freckles, and it also prevents the formation of pus, making it an excellent agent for removing blackheads. Papain, an enzyme of papaya, softens tissues rich in protein.

Papaya juice is not suitable for use in creams or lotions as it is very strong and can irritate even the most tolerant of skins.

Papaya mask

4 tbsp papaya juice (if this
 is unobtainable, you can
 press it yourself)
50 ml (3 tbsp) distilled
 water
50 ml (3 tbsp) camomile
 tea
oatmeal

Press the papaya juice out
of a papaya fruit – this pres-
ents no problem to an electric fruit press, but if one is
not available, there are two
other ways of doing it:

1.

Cut the papaya in half and
rub honey into the two
halves. Leave them for
some time before cutting
the papaya into cubes and
pressing out the juice with
the aid of a sieve.

2.

Peel the papaya and grate
it with a grater. Place the
grated fruit in a silk cloth
and squeeze hard to pro-
duce the juice.

Mix the papaya juice
with the distilled water and
the camomile tea, then
gently heat the mixture.
Add enough oatmeal
(crushed hulled oats) to
produce a smooth, easily
workable paste. Apply the
papaya mask to moist skin
and leave in place for ten
minutes at most. Rinse

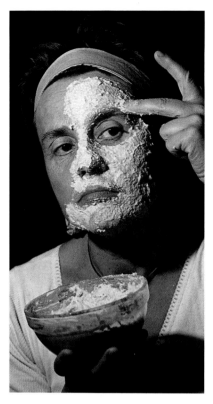

away thoroughly, being
careful not to rub the face
too much.

A papaya mask softens
the skin, and removes
dead cells and blackheads.
On no account must it be
used on sensitive skin.

Painting with papaya juice

Paint the face with the
juice and leave it on for no
more than five minutes.
Avoid the area around the
eyes. Rinse carefully with
lukewarm water, and then
with cold water.

Papaya juice can be
used to paint any part of
the body where the skin
feels dry and rough; it has
a deep-going effect. On no
account should people
with allergies or sensitive,
easily irritated skin use papaya juice for painting,
however.

Strawberry

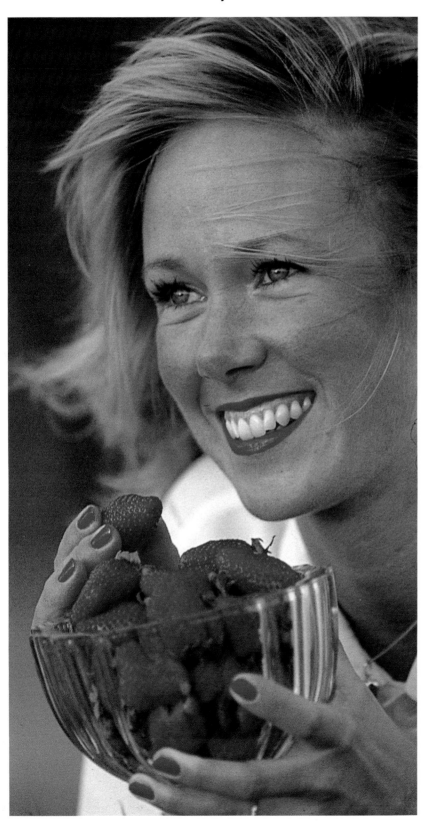

Strawberries are cleansing and astringent, and should be used first and foremost on oily skin or skin with large pores. By reducing the size of the pores, strawberries control excess oil around the nose, on the forehead and on the chin. It is essential that strawberries used in face masks or creams should be unsprayed: strawberries are among the berries that are subjected to most chemical treatment of all fruits, and if there is one thing above all else which leads to allergies, it is chemical treatment to protect fruit from insects and plant diseases.

Face mask for tired and jaded skin

5 strawberries
2 tbsp yoghurt
2 tsp honey
almond flour (finely ground sweet almonds)

A refreshing and astringent mask which should not be used on dry skin or skin susceptible to allergy.

Rinse the strawberries thoroughly in hot water and remove all blemishes, then mash them together with the yoghurt and mix in the honey. Add almond flour to form a smooth, easily spread paste. Leave the strawberry mask in place for about ten minutes, then rinse off with lukewarm water.

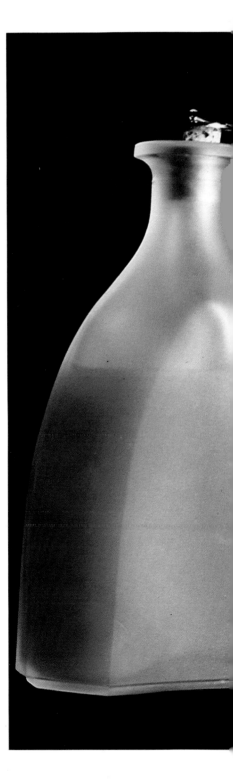

Strawberry lotion for oily skin

5 tbsp fresh strawberry leaves
100 ml (6 tbsp) distilled water
100 ml (6 tbsp) rose water
1 tsp borax
1 pinch sodium benzoate, if desired

An astringent face lotion which can also be used as an after-shave.

Boil the distilled water and pour it over the well-washed strawberry leaves, and leave to draw in a container with a lid for at least five hours. Heat the rose water gently and dissolve the borax in it, and also the preservative if required. Strain off the liquid from the strawberry leaves and add the rose water to it, shake well, and pour the face lotion into a thoroughly cleaned bottle. Keep in a cold place.

A strawberry lotion that is different

20 g (3/4 oz) cocoa butter
6 tbsp almond oil
5 tbsp glycerol
8 tbsp pure strawberry juice
2 tbsp distilled water
1 pinch agar-agar
1 pinch sodium benzoate, if desired
1 teaspoon borax

This lotion freshens, firms and nourishes, but it can be risky to use it on allergic skin: as is well known, strawberries are very "strong".

Melt the cocoa butter and almond oil together in a water-bath, stirring gently until the mixture is clear and smooth. Meanwhile, heat up the distilled water together with the pure strawberry juice, adding the borax and also the sodium benzoate if desired. Stir the glycerol carefully into the oil mixture, and keep stirring until all the glycerol has combined with the fats. Then take one pinch of agar-agar and whisk it into the strawberry juice. Whisk vigorously with an electric whisk so that no lumps are formed, then quickly remove the oil mixture from the water-bath and whisk into it the strawberry jelly. Whisk vigorously with an electric whisk for a long time, and continue until the mixture has cooled down completely before pouring the strawberry lotion into a thoroughly cleaned jar, which should be kept in a cool, dark place.

1. Mix hot distilled water with fresh, pure strawberry juice.

2. Whisk in a pinch of agar-agar.

3. Add the oil mixture. Whisk vigorously.

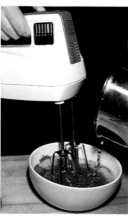
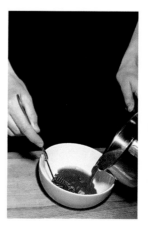
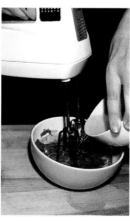

Rose hip

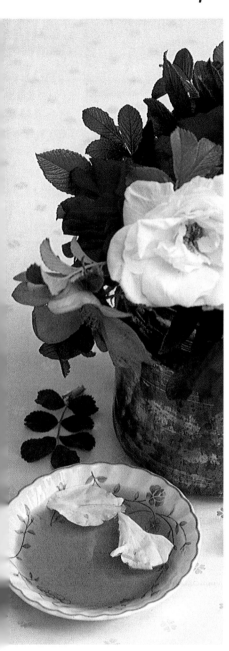

Rose hips are rich in vitamin C and very good for the skin, refreshing it and endowing it with a slight radiance.

Eye wash to prevent bags forming

1 tbsp dried rose hips
100 ml (6 tbsp) distilled water

Boil the water and pour it over the rose hips, then allow it to draw for at least an hour. Strain the eye wash and use it for bathing swollen eyelids. It is also useful for combating bags under the eyes. The best results are obtained by soaking a little pad of gauze in the eye wash, and applying it like a compress.

Face lotion

4 tbsp crushed dried rose hips
200 ml (7 fl oz) distilled water
1 tsp apple-cider vinegar
4 tsp almond oil
2 teaspoons granulated lecithin

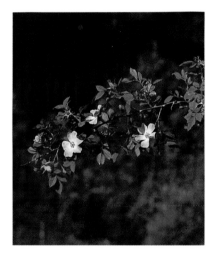

Rose-hip face lotion is refreshing, and the apple-cider vinegar restores the correct pH value to the skin.

Boil the water and pour it over the rose hips, allowing it to draw for at least an hour before straining through thin muslin. Heat the almond oil in a water-bath, add the lecithin and stir gently until the granules have dissolved. Remove the dish from the water-bath and heat the strained rose-hip water. Add the apple-cider vinegar to the warm rose-hip water. Then pour the rose-hip water extremely slowly into the oil mixture and whisk vigorously with an electric whisk. Keep on whisking until the face water has cooled completely. Pour into a thoroughly cleaned bottle, and keep in a refrigerator. Shake the bottle before using.

Cocoa

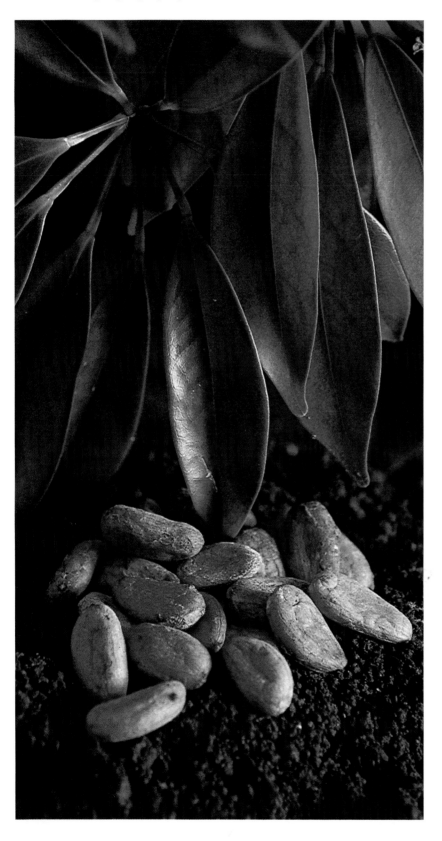

Cocoa butter is obtained from roasted cocoa beans, and is a firm, yellowish-white fat often used as the base for creams and lotions. It is used so widely because of its moisturizing properties.

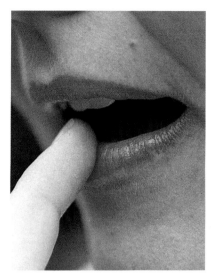
Dry lips need a lip salve regularly to keep them soft. This is simple to make.

Cocoa lotion

15 g (1/2 oz) cocoa butter
1 tbsp lanolin
125 ml (7 1/2 tbsp) wheat-germ oil
1 teaspoon honey
3 tbsp distilled water
1 pinch sodium benzoate, if desired

Cocoa lotion can be used all over the body. It is moisturizing, and makes the skin supple.

Melt together the cocoa butter, lanolin, oil and honey in a water-bath. When the oil mixture is completely smooth and homogeneous, and everything has fused together, you can remove the dish from the water-bath. Heat up the distilled water quickly, and if a preservative is to be used, dissolve it in the water. Add the water to the oil mixture, one spoon at a time, while whisking vigorously with an electric whisk. Continue whisking for some considerable time after all the water has been added; when the cream is lukewarm and stable, the whisking can be done with a small balloon whisk. Keep the cocoa lotion in a cool, dry place.

Lip salve

5 g (1 tsp) beeswax
4 tbsp cocoa butter
1 tsp coconut oil
1 drop fragrant oil (can be omitted)

An excellent lip salve for dry and chapped lips.

Melt the wax in a water-bath, then add the cocoa butter and stir until the mixture is smooth. Add the coconut oil and, if desired, the fragrant oil. Remove the dish from the water-bath and whisk vigorously with a small balloon whisk until the salve has cooled down completely. Spoon it into a thoroughly cleaned jar, and keep in a cool place.

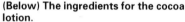
(Below) The ingredients for the cocoa lotion.

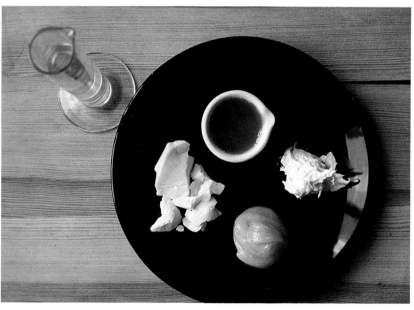

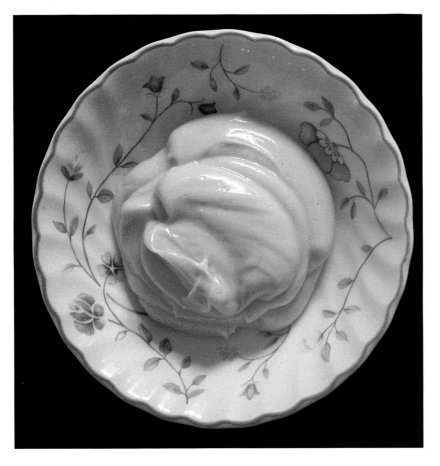

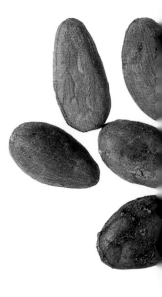

Healing cream with cocoa butter

5 g (1 tsp) beeswax or
   white wax
15 g (1/2 oz) cocoa butter
2 tbsp almond oil
2 tbsp glycerol
5 tbsp elderflower water
4 tbsp wheat-germ oil
3 tbsp distilled water
1 pinch sodium benzoate,
   if desired
fragrant oil, if required

Melt the wax, cocoa butter
and oils in a water-bath.
Meanwhile, heat up the
liquid – the elderflower
mixed with the distilled
water – and if a preserv-
ative is desired, it should
be dissolved in the liquid at
this point. When the oil mixture has fused completely
and is smooth, stir in the
glycerol. Remove the dish
from the water-bath and
add the liquid, one spoon at
a time, while whisking
vigorously with an electric
whisk. Keep on whisking
until the cream is luke-
warm, at which point the
electric whisk can be
replaced by a small balloon
whisk; continue beating
until the cream has cooled
down completely. If a
fragrant oil is required, add
it now. If necessary, the
elderflower water can be replaced by distilled water
alone.

Elderflower water – see
page 80.

Spoon the cream into a
thoroughly cleaned jar, and
keep in a cool, dark place.

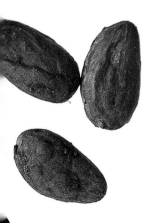

Sun lotion with cocoa butter

25 g (1 oz) cocoa butter
5 tbsp sesame oil
1 tbsp granulated lecithin
2 tsp glycerol
2 tbsp lavender extract,
 camomile extract, or just
 distilled water
2 tbsp aloe jelly
1 pinch sodium benzoate,
 if desired

Heat the sesame oil in a water-bath, then add the granulated lecithin, stirring or agitating constantly with a small balloon whisk until all the lecithin has dissolved into the oil. Heat the liquid, i.e. the extract or simply water, and if a preservative is desired, it should be added to the liquid at this point. Add the glycerol to the oil mixture and stir quite vigorously. Remove the dish from the water-bath and carefully add the liquid, one spoon at a time, whisking constantly with an electric whisk. After a while, add the aloe jelly one spoon at a time, still whisking vigorously. Keep on whisking until the lotion, which should be relatively thick in consistency, is quite smooth and has "set". When the lotion has cooled down completely, pour it into a thoroughly cleaned jar, and store in a cool, dark place.

Camomile extract – see page 56.

Lavender extract – add 3 tbsp dried lavender to 125 ml (7 1/2 tbsp) distilled water. Boil the water, and pour it over the flowers, then allow the mixture to stand for rather more than an hour. Strain off the flowers, and use the extract in creams and lotions.

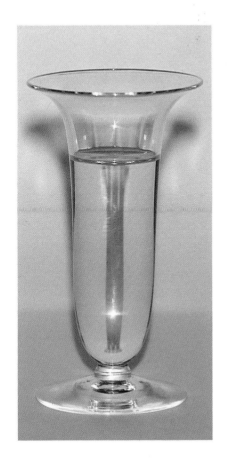

Sesame oil.

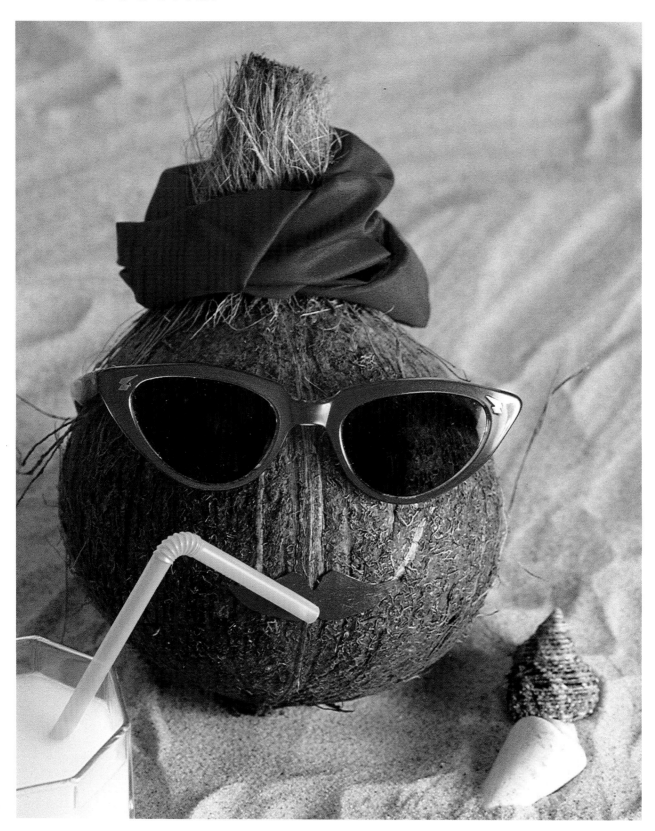

Coconut oil, or coconut butter – they are in fact the same thing – is a good skin-softener. Coconut contains a lot of phosphorus, and endows the skin and hair with a delicate radiance. Coconut oil is good for chapped lips and blemished skin, and coconut butter is a moisturizer.

Melted coconut butter is the same as coconut oil, then, and coconut butter can normally be obtained from large grocery stores.

Face mask with coconut milk

100 ml (6 tbsp) coconut milk
2 tsp glycerol
200 ml (7 fl oz) oatmeal

This coconut mask provides the skin with so much moisture, the skin is shocked into a reaction; the abrasive effect of the oatmeal induces an additional softening effect.

Heat the coconut milk gently, and add the glycerol; whisk to form a smooth mixture, then add the oatmeal and work the resultant mass into a smooth paste. If necessary, a little more coconut milk or a little distilled water can be added. Apply the face mask and leave in place for about thirty minutes before rinsing away with lukewarm water.

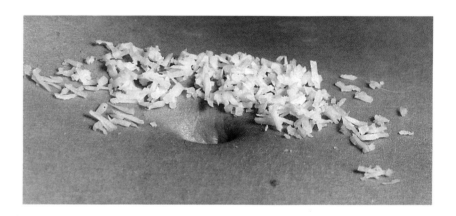

Scrub mask for the whole body

300 ml (1/2 pt) shredded coconut (preferably fresh)
200 ml (7 fl oz) finely shredded sweet almonds
200 ml (7 fl oz) oatmeal
3 tbsp honey
distilled water

This effective mask has a softening effect on all types of skin.

Mix all the ingredients and add the heated distilled water until the mixture is smooth. Apply the mask to the face and other parts of the body where the skin feels rough and chapped. Leave it in place for about half an hour, then massage it away with rotary movements before rinsing with lukewarm water. Apply a gentle moisturizing cream.

Cleansing lotion with coconut

4 tbsp coconut oil
75 ml (4 1/2 tbsp) almond
  oil
2 tbsp glycerol
1 tbsp granulated lecithin
5 tbsp distilled water
1/2 tsp borax
1 pinch sodium benzoate,
  if desired

Heat the almond oil in a water-bath, add the granulated lecithin and allow it to dissolve completely in the almond oil before adding the coconut oil. Meanwhile, heat up the distilled water and dissolve the borax in it: if a preservative is desired, now is the time to dissolve it in the water. Add the glycerol to the oil mixture and remove the dish from the water-bath. Carefully add the hot water one spoon at a time, whisking constantly with an electric whisk. Continue whisking until the lotion has "whitened" (emulsified). When the cream is lukewarm, you can continue beating with a small balloon whisk – but be sure to continue whisking until the lotion has cooled down completely.

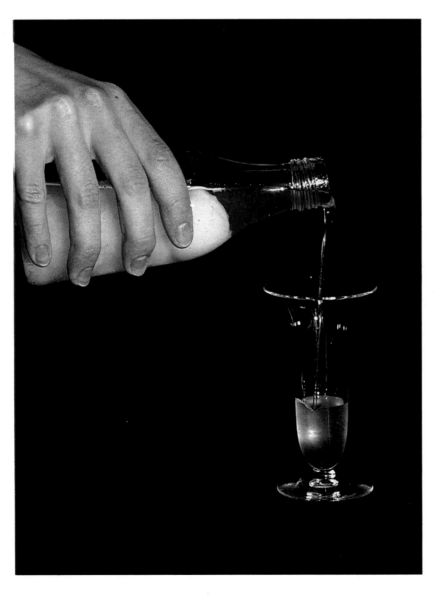

Lip salve with coconut

5 g (1 tsp) coconut butter
2 tsp coconut oil
5 drops glycerol

Lip salve with coconut gives the lips a slight radiance.

Melt all the ingredients in a water-bath, whisking all the time with a small balloon whisk. When the mixture is clear and smooth, remove the dish from the water-bath and continue whisking until the lip salve has cooled down completely and hardened. If you keep the lip salve in a refrigerator, it will become extremely hard: it is thus advisable to try and roll the salve into a stick before putting it into the refrigerator, so that it is easier to apply.

Coconut oil helps dry skin.

Almond

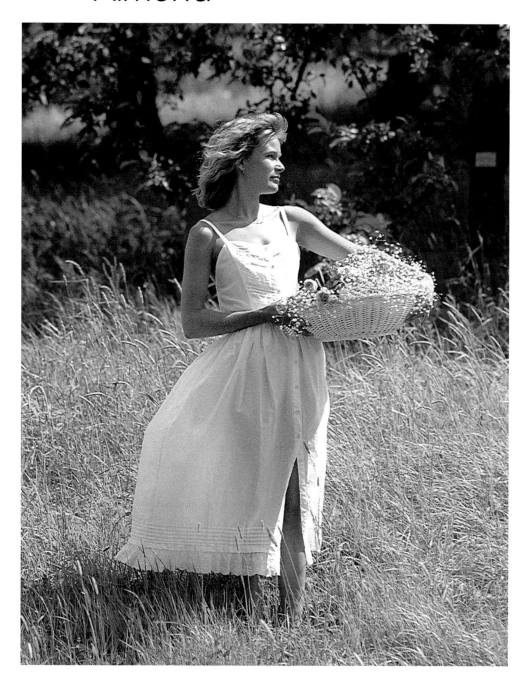

Crushed sweet almonds and almond oil are very beneficial for the skin. Almond also has a high level of acidity and thus can easily remove wrinkled or dead layers of skin. Almond oil is often used as a base in creams and lotions, and when warm it is also a simple and effective cleansing agent, especially for dry skin. Almond also has a healing effect.

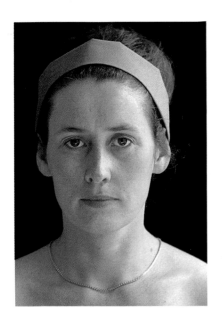

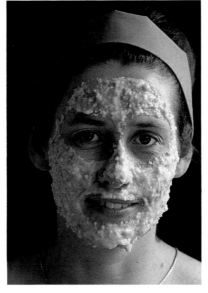

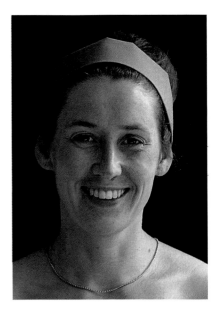

Almond mask for blackheads and dead skin cells

75 g (2 1/2 oz) scalded and peeled sweet almonds
1/2 mashed ripe tomato
distilled water

Reduce the almonds in a mixer, then mix with the mashed tomato and distilled water to form a fine paste. Apply mask and leave in place for fifteen minutes. Remove by rubbing.

Blackheads can be steamed away easily after treatment with an almond mask, and dead skin cells disappear automatically as you rub the mask off.

Mask for flushed and nervous skin

75 g (2 1/2 oz) scalded and peeled almonds
2 tsp glycerol
4 tbsp yoghurt
distilled water or camomile extract

This mask soothes nervous skin and removes blemishes and flushed skin.

Reduce the almonds in a mixer, then heat the glycerol and yoghurt in a water-bath and mix the result with the ground almonds. Heat up the distilled water, about 100 ml (6 tbsp) to start with, and add it while quite hot, then work the mixture into a smooth paste, adding more water if necessary. Apply the face mask while it is still a little warm, and leave it for about fifteen minutes.

Mask for dry and jaded skin

1/2 egg white
1 tbsp honey
60 g (2 1/4 oz) scalded and peeled sweet almonds
distilled water

This mask is cleansing and nourishing.

Reduce the almonds in a mixer and add a little distilled water until the mixture looks like a finely grained, thick gruel, then add the honey and egg white and whisk vigorously for a short while. Apply the face mask immediately and leave in place for at least twenty minutes before rinsing off with lukewarm water.

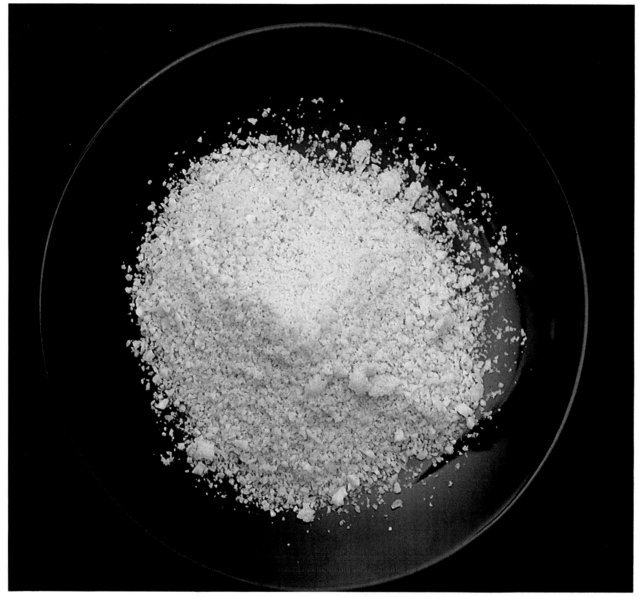

Crushed almonds.

Simple almond lotion

50 g (2 oz) scalded and
   peeled almonds
3/4 litre (1 1/2 pt) rose water
2 tsp honey
1 tsp borax
1 pinch sodium benzoate,
   if desired

Almond lotion nourishes tired and jaded skin, and also has a healing effect.

Mix the almonds and the rose water in a mixer: the mixture should be runny and very finely pulverized when it is ready. Strain the almond mixture through a fine muslin, then heat up the almond lotion before adding the borax and honey, and also, if desired, the preservative. Shake the mixture well, and pour into a thoroughly cleaned bottle. Keep in a cool place

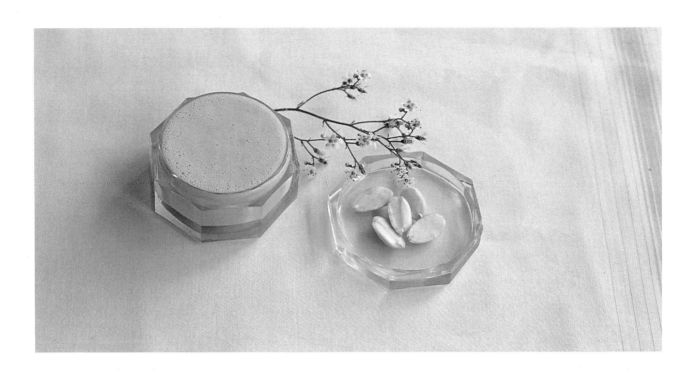

Cleansing cream with almond oil

10 g (1 tsp) white wax
1 1/2 tbsp glycerol
125 ml (7 1/2 tbsp) almond oil
3 tbsp rose water
1 pinch sodium benzoate, if desired

Melt the wax and almond oil together in a water-bath, stirring with a small balloon whisk until everything has melted and the mixture is clear and smooth. Meanwhile, heat up the rose water, and if a preservative is required, dissolve it in the warm rose water. Add the glycerol to the oil mixture and stir until the mixture is homogeneous again. Remove the dish from the water-bath and carefully add the hot rose water one spoon at a time while whisking vigorously with an electric whisk. When all the water has been added, continue whisking vigorously until the cream is lukewarm and stabilized. A small balloon whisk can now be used to beat the cream until it has cooled down completely. Use a spoon to transfer the cream into a thoroughly cleaned jar, and keep it in a cool, dark place.

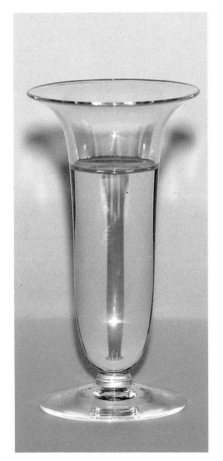

Almond oil.

Simple almond milk

300 ml (1/2 pt) sweet almonds
50 ml (3 tbsp) thick cream
200 ml (7 fl oz) milk
1/2 tsp borax
1 pinch sodium benzoate, if desired

Use almond milk either as a lotion prior to applying a night cream, or as a rapid refreshener for tired and jaded skin.

Scald and peel the almonds, and reduce them in a mixer. Meanwhile, heat the milk and cream together with the borax, and add the preservative if required. The milk mixture should not be allowed to boil. Add the crushed almonds to the milk mixture, and allow to simmer under a lid for several hours. Squeeze the almond milk through a thin silk cloth, allow to cool somewhat, then pour it into a thoroughly cleaned bottle.

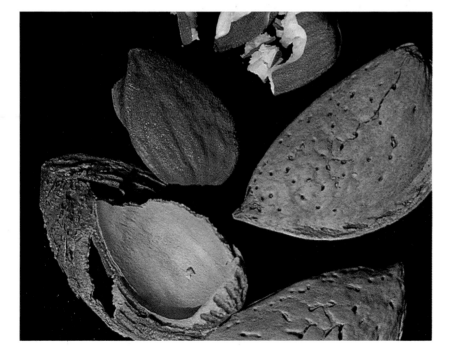

Simple night cream with almond oil

100 ml (6 tbsp) almond oil
3 tbsp lanolin
2 tbsp glycerol
75 ml (4 1/2 tbsp) rose water
1 pinch sodium benzoate, if desired
some drops genuine fragrant oil, optional

Melt the almond oil and the lanolin in a water-bath, stirring gently until all the lanolin has dissolved and the mixture is smooth and fine. Meanwhile, heat up the rose water, and if a preservative is required, add it to the hot rose water. Then add the glycerol to the oil mixture and stir for a while before removing the dish from the water-bath and carefully adding the hot rose water, a spoon at a time, while whisking vigorously with an electric whisk. Keep on whisking until the cream is almost cold, at which point you can use a small balloon whisk to beat it gently. Carry on whisking until the cream has cooled down completely, then use a spoon to transfer it into a thoroughly cleaned jar and keep it in a cool, dark place.

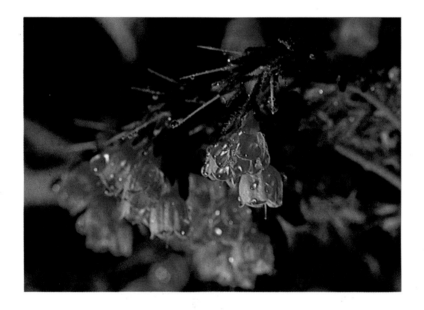

Comfrey. Both leaves and roots can be used in creams and lotions.

Camomile

Marigold

Yarrow

Comfrey

Fennel

Rosemary

Nettle

Rose

Aloe Vera

Witch-hazel

Elder

Camomile

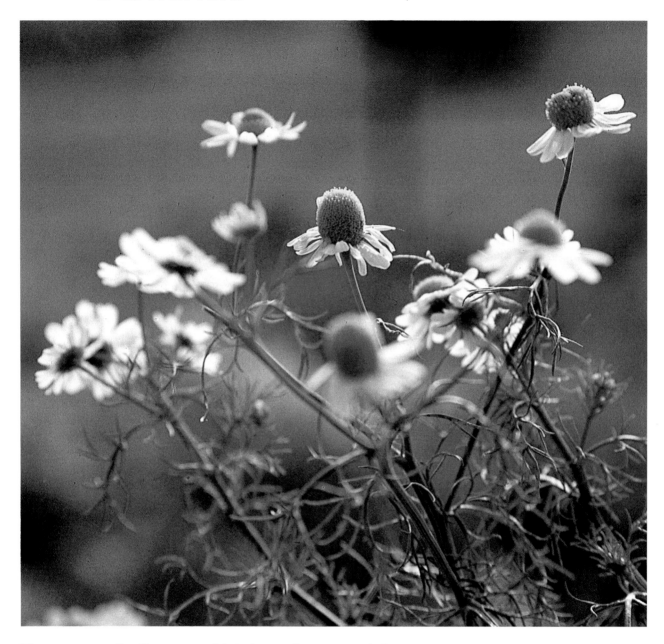

The camomile flower, which is really a weed, is very useful for skin care. The flower has a strengthening and cleansing effect, and soothes nervous or irritated skin. Camomile is a common wild flower, and it is mainly the flowers that are used for cosmetics. Be choosy about where you pick your camomile flowers, and avoid plants which may be affected by industrial or traffic pollution.

Face mask with camomile

2 tbsp camomile
3 tbsp almond flour (finely
   ground sweet almonds)
3 tbsp water
2 tbsp yoghurt
1 tbsp honey

Camomile is suitable for all types of skin. This mask is cleansing and soothing, and has a gently abrasive effect due to the ground almonds.

Mix all the ingredients carefully; an electric mixer is most appropriate. Apply the face mask and leave in place for at least half an hour before rinsing off with lukewarm water.

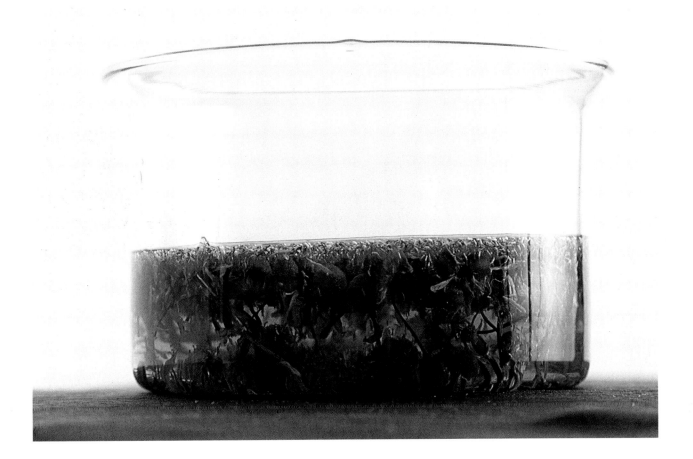

Camomile oil

1 dried camomile flower
200 ml (7 fl oz) almond oil
100 ml (6 tbsp) thistle oil
2 tbsp honey

Camomile oil can be used all over the body, and is very good for lifeless and jaded skin.

Heat the oils and the honey in a water-bath, then add the camomile flower and allow to stand over heat for about half an hour.

Remove from the heat and keep the oil mixture in a container with a lid for twenty-four hours before straining off the camomile flower and pouring the oil into a thoroughly cleaned jar. Keep the oil in a refrigerator.

Camomile cream

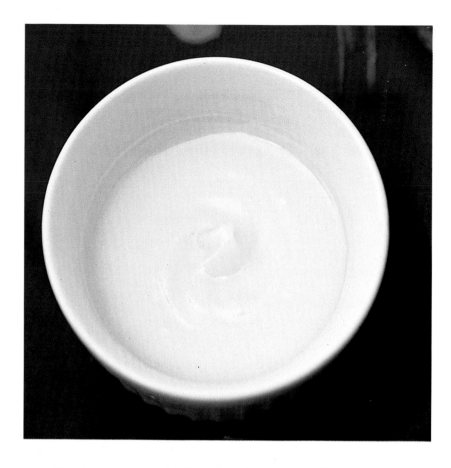

Camomile cream has many uses, being both healing and cleansing. It has a soothing effect on nervous skin.

10 g (2 tsp) beeswax or
　　white wax
5 tbsp almond oil
1 tbsp wheatgerm oil
2 tbsp glycerol
2 tbsp distilled water
4 tbsp camomile extract
　　(see below for
　　proportions)
1 tbsp honey
sodium benzoate,
　　if desired

Melt the wax and oil together in a water-bath, stirring gently with a small balloon whisk until a smooth, clear mixture is formed. Meanwhile, heat the distilled water together with the camomile extract, then add the glycerol and honey to the oil mixture and whisk gently until it is once more clear and smooth. Remove the dish from the water-bath and add the warm liquid very carefully, whisking vigorously all the while – an electric whisk is essential here. Continue whisking until the cream has "set" and is cool rather than warm – at which point you may go over to a small balloon whisk, and keep beating until the cream has cooled down completely. Use a spoon to transfer it into containers, which should be kept in a cool, dark place.

Camomile extract is made by adding 2 tbsp camomile flowers to 100 ml (6 tbsp) distilled water. Boil the water and pour it over the flowers, then allow to stand for at least three hours, preferably in a container with a lid. Strain off the flowers, and use the extract in creams and lotions.

Marigold

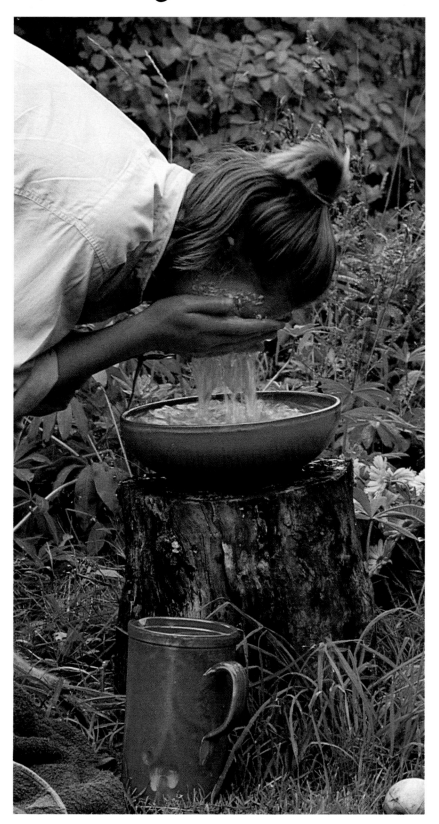

Marigold is a very versatile agent in the field of cosmetics. It softens and cleanses, heals sores, is antiseptic, and hence is good for inflamed skin and acne. The flower itself is suitable for rubbing into swellings like the ones caused by wasp stings: it eases the throbbing pain considerably. Marigolds are very common in gardens, and well-stocked health food shops always have dried marigold.

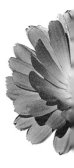

Marigold mask

100 ml (6 tbsp) marigold
   petals (dried or fresh)
4 tbsp yoghurt
1 tbsp granulated lecithin
4 tbsp oatmeal
50 ml (3 tbsp)
   distilled water

A marigold mask is very refreshing; it heals any inflam-
mation and cleanses skin
affected by acne.
   Boil the water and pour
over the chopped petals.
Mix in the yoghurt, oatmeal
and lecithin, stirring vigorously. Apply the mixture
while it is still lukewarm.
Leave it on for half an hour
before rinsing off with lukewarm water.

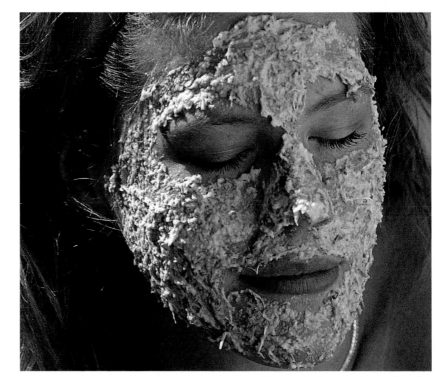

The marigold mask is excellent for inflamed skin.

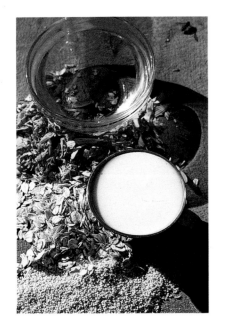

Face lotion with marigold

100 ml (6 tbsp) fresh marigold
2 tbsp dried camomile flowers
400 ml (3/4 pt) distilled water
1/2 tsp borax
1 pinch sodium benzoate, if desired

Face lotion with marigold and camomile is both cleansing
and healing. It revitalizes tired skin, and soothes nervous
blemishes.
   Cut up the marigolds and mix them with the dried
camomile flowers, then boil the water and pour it over the
floral mixture. Pour the infusion, leaves and all, into a bottle
and cork it well. Leave the bottle in a light place for two
days. After twenty-four hours, add the borax and shake
vigorously. If a preservative is desired, it should be
dissolved in a little hot water and added together with the
borax. After two more days, strain the face lotion and transfer it into a thoroughly cleaned bottle, which is then kept in
a cool place.

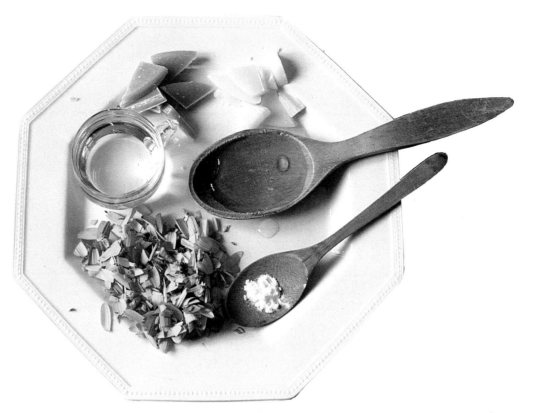

Marigold cream

10 g (1 tsp) white wax
3 tbsp almond oil
2 tbsp wheat-germ oil
1 tbsp glycerol
4 – 5 tbsp marigold extract
(see below for
proportions)
1/2 tsp borax
1 pinch sodium benzoate,
if desired

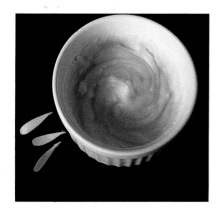

This cream is suitable for all types of skin. It nourishes, tones, and acts as a moisturizer.

Melt the wax and oils in a water-bath and stir with a small balloon whisk until the mixture is smooth and clear. Heat the marigold extract until it reaches approximately the same temperature as the oil mixture; do not let it boil. Add the borax to the marigold extract, and the sodium benzoate, if any. Add the glycerol to the oil mixture, and stir gently. Remove the dish from the water-bath and add the marigold extract, one spoon at a time, while whisking vigorously with an electric whisk. Continue whisking after all the liquid has been added, until the cream has cooled almost completely: at this point, the electric whisk may be replaced by a small balloon whisk. When it is quite cool, pour it into a thoroughly cleaned jar, and keep in a cool place.

Marigold extract is made by mixing 75 ml (4 1/2 tbsp) cut marigold petals and 125 ml (7 1/2 tbsp) distilled water. Boil the water and pour it over the petals, then let the infusion stand in a container with a lid to draw for three hours. Strain, and use in creams and lotions.

Yarrow

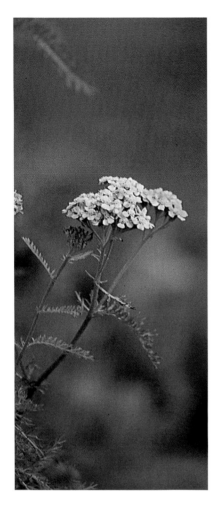

Face lotion with yarrow

200 ml (7 fl oz) distilled water
2 tbsp dried yarrow
1 tsp almond oil
1/2 tsp borax
1 tsp glycerol

This face lotion has a drying effect. If your skin is very oily and you want a face lotion which has a marked drying effect, you should omit both the almond oil and the glycerol.

Boil the water and pour it over the yarrow, then add the glycerol and almond oil and whisk until cool. Add the borax powder, and keep whisking until it has dissolved completely. Strain off the flowers when the face lotion is cold, then pour into a thoroughly cleaned bottle and keep in a cool place. Shake the bottle before use.

Yarrow mask for acne and excessively oily skin

3 tbsp yarrow extract (see below for proportions)
3 tbsp kaolin (powder)
1 tbsp yoghurt

Mix all the ingredients to form a smooth paste. Apply the mask evenly over the face, but avoid the area around the eyes. Leave in place for fifteen minutes, then rinse away with lukewarm water.

Yarrow extract is made by mixing 1 1/2 tbsp dried yarrow and 100 ml (6 tbsp) distilled water. Boil the water and pour it over the flowers, then leave to draw for about an hour. This yarrow mask has a marked drying effect, and should only be used by people with really oily skin.

In both the above recipes, the yarrow can be replaced by sage, which has characteristics similar to those of yarrow. Sage is not as strong as yarrow, however, and can therefore be used on normal skin.

Yarrow is a common wild flower. It flowers in late summer, and should be picked immediately after the flowers have opened. Only the flowers are used. Yarrow is a powerful astringent, and hence effective for large pores. It also has a drying effect and should therefore be used first and foremost by people with oily skins.

Comfrey

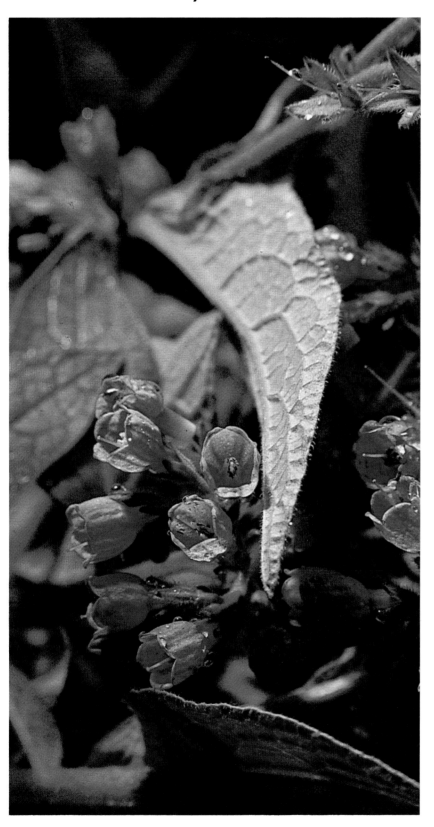

Comfrey often grows in large beds on the banks of ditches, and in recent years has acquired considerable importance for skin care. Analysis has shown that it contains allantoin, a very important substance for promoting the growth of skin cells. Comfrey can be grown in all parts of the country. The leaves or roots are used in creams and face lotions.

Comfrey has a healing, slightly astringent and softening effect. It is also very effective for chapped skin.

Comfrey mask

2 tbsp dried comfrey
   leaves (4 tbsp if fresh)
2 tsp honey
1 tbsp glycerol
50 ml (3 tbsp) distilled
   water
arrowroot flour

This comfrey mask is a genuine super-moisturizer. It has a softening effect, and livens up tired skin.

Chop the comfrey leaves or reduce in a mixer, then boil the water and pour it over them and add the glycerol and honey. Stir, and add sufficient arrowroot flour to make an easily worked paste. Apply the face mask and leave in place for about fifteen minutes before rinsing off with luke-warm water.

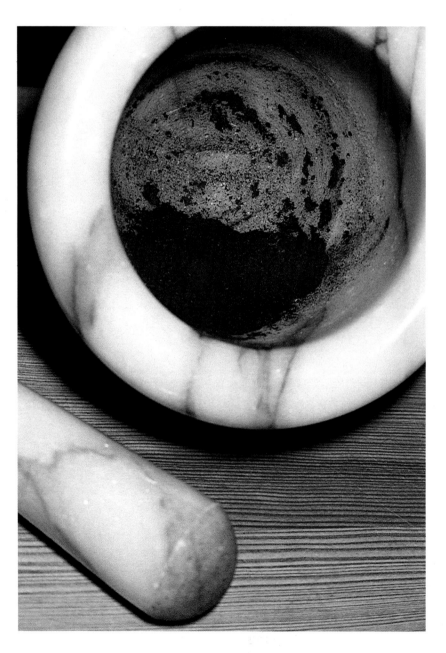

Clean the comfrey root well, then grind it to a fine powder.

Comfrey water

1 tbsp crushed comfrey
   root
800 ml (1 1/2 pt) distilled
   water
1 teaspoon borax

Comfrey water is used for bathing the face, or as a softening agent in face masks, instead of distilled water.

Boil the crushed comfrey in the water for about fifteen minutes, then allow to draw for at least three hours. Strain through thin muslin, or a coffee filter, then heat a little and add the borax. Transfer the comfrey water into a thoroughly cleaned bottle and keep in a cold place.

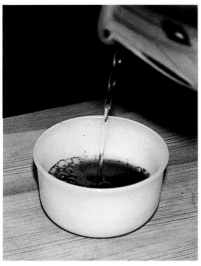

1. Pour the boiling water over the powdered root.

Comfrey cream

15 g (1/2 oz) cocoa butter
5 g (1/2 tsp) white wax
1 tbsp glycerol
4 tbsp almond oil
3 tbsp comfrey extract (see
   below for proportions)
2 tbsp distilled water
1 pinch sodium benzoate,
   if desired

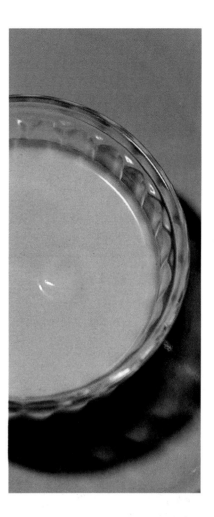

2. Add glycerol to the oil mixture. Mix in the comfrey extract carefully and whisk until it is cool.

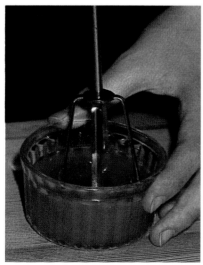

This is a very benevolent and healing cream for all kinds of skin.

Heat the cocoa butter and oil in a water-bath, stirring until the mixture is smooth and clear. Meanwhile, mix the comfrey extract and distilled water in a saucepan and heat to about the same temperature as the oil mixture. If a preservative is desired, it should be dissolved at this stage in the liquid. Add the glycerol to the oil mixture, and stir. Remove the dish from the water-bath and add the hot liquid carefully, one spoon at a time. Whisk with an electric whisk until the cream is lukewarm, then use a small balloon whisk until it has cooled completely.

Comfrey extract is made by mixing 2 1/2 teaspoons comfrey root (crushed) and 100 ml (6 tbsp) distilled water. Pour the boiling water over the powdered root and allow to draw for one hour. Strain.

Fennel

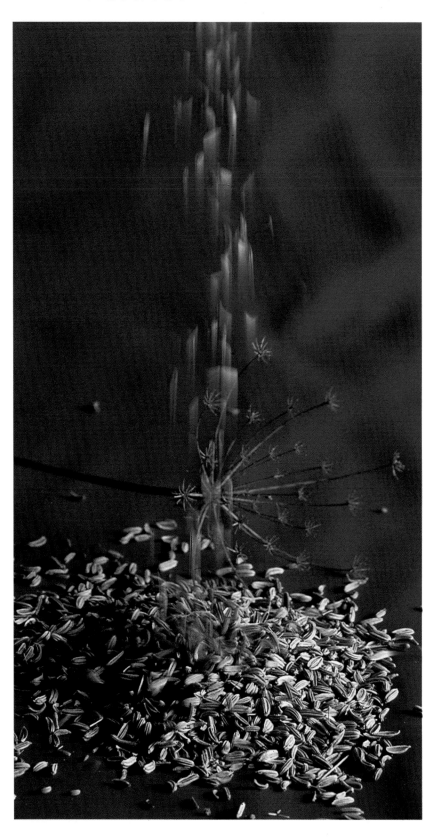

Fennel is very effective with tired and lifeless skin. It also removes impurities, such as blackheads and excess grease particles in the skin. Fennel has also been shown to have a healing and soothing effect on eczema.

Fennel cream

5 g (1/2 tsp) beeswax
15 g (1/2 oz) cocoa butter
3 tbsp almond oil
1 tbsp glycerol
1 tsp honey
4 tbsp fennel water (for
    proportions see below)
1 pinch sodium benzoate,
    if desired

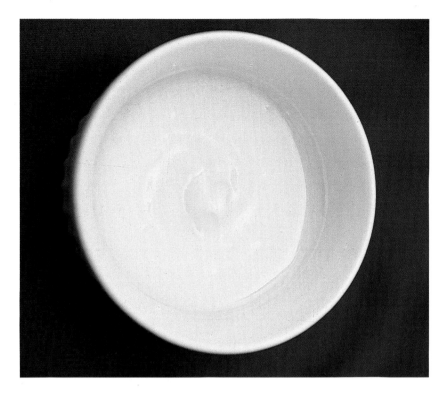

Fennel cream should be used on lifeless and wrinkled skin all over the body.

Melt the beeswax, almond oil and cocoa butter in a water-bath, then add the honey after a little while. Stir constantly with a small balloon whisk until the oil mixture is smooth and clear. Heat the fennel water, but do not allow it to boil. If sodium benzoate is required, it should be dissolved in the hot water. Remove the oil mixture from the water-bath and add the glycerol, stirring all the time, and then add the fennel water while whisking with an electric whisk. Continue whisking until the cream has ''whitened'' (emulsified), after which you can continue whisking with a small balloon whisk until the cream has cooled down completely. Keep in a cool, dark place.

Anti-wrinkle mask

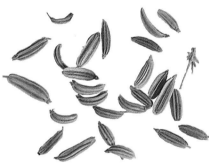

2 tbsp glycerol
8 tbsp fennel water (see
    below for proportions)
100 g (3 1/2 oz) kaolin
    (in powder form)

This mask deep-cleans and smooths.

Heat the glycerol in a water-bath, add the fennel water and stir vigorously. Mix in the kaolin, one spoon at a time, and continue to beat the paste until it feels smooth and fine. Apply the face mask from below, starting at the neck and chin and working up to the forehead. Leave the mask in place for fifteen minutes, then rinse with lukewarm water and wait for about half an hour before using any moisturizing cream.

Make the fennel water for the mask by mixing 2 tbsp of fennel seed with 200 ml (7 fl oz) distilled water. Boil the water and pour it over the seed; allow it to draw for twenty-four hours, then strain.

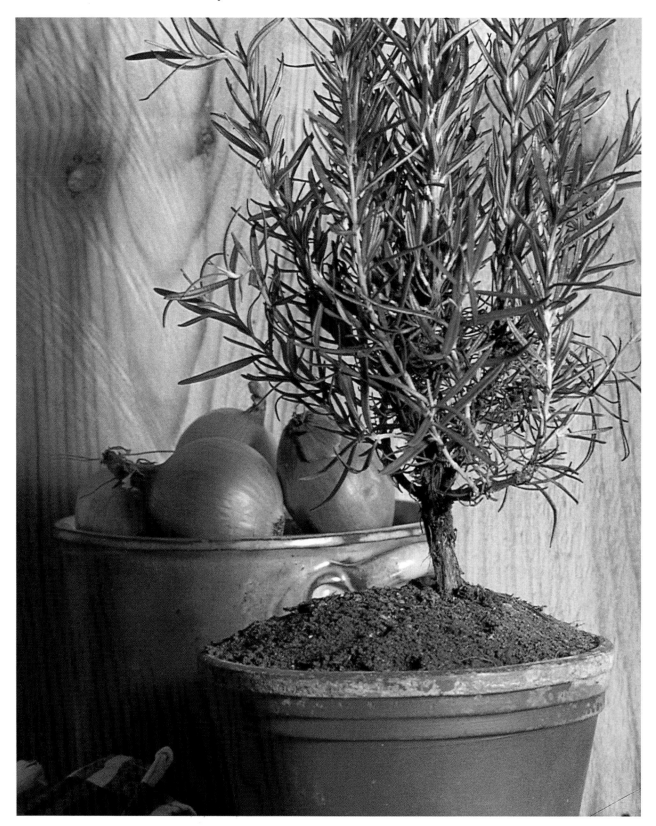

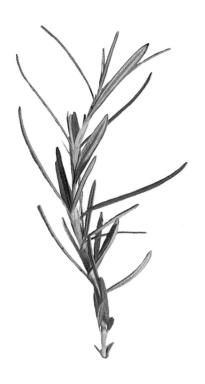

Rosemary water

200 ml (7 1/2 fl oz) distilled water
2 tbsp dried rosemary (4 tbsp if fresh)
1 tsp almond or groundnut oil
1 pinch sodium benzoate

Rosemary water can be used as an after-shave. As a face lotion, it should be patted into the skin after cleaning at night. Shake the bottle before use.

Boil the water and pour it over the rosemary leaves, cover with a lid, and leave to draw for at least three hours. Add the oil, and whisk gently for a while before straining and pouring the rosemary water into a thoroughly cleaned bottle.

Rosemary is used primarily in face lotions and masks as far as cosmetics are concerned. It is astringent and helps the circulation.

Rosemary mask

3 tbsp kaolin clay
1 1/2 tbsp rosemary extract (see below for proportions)
2 tsp glycerol

Mix all the ingredients in a basin, stirring to form a smooth paste; if more liquid is needed, add distilled water until the desired consistency is attained. Apply the face mask, avoiding the area around the eyes, and leave in place for about twenty minutes. Remove the mask by rinsing with luke-warm water. It cleanses in depth, has an abrasive effect, and smooths out irregularities.

Rosemary extract is made by mixing 1 tbsp dried leaves and 75 ml (4 1/2 tbsp) distilled water. Boil the water and pour it over the herb, then leave to draw for three hours. If fresh rosemary is used, take 2 tbsp for the same amount of water.

Nettles

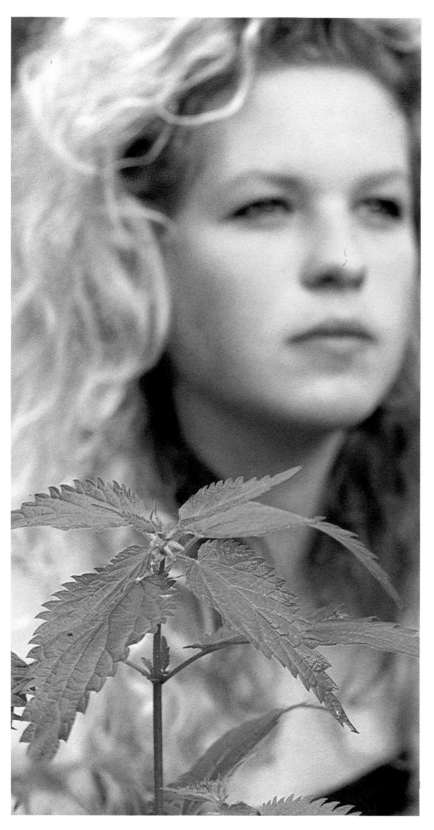

Nettles are suitable for all types of skin, and have a cleansing, healing effect. Nettles contain both antihistamines and sulphur, which makes them especially suitable for the dry, sensitive skin caused by eczema. Nettles are also effective treatment for other allergic rashes, and soothe nervous complexions with superficial blood vessels and blemishes. The secretion of fat is reduced by nettle treatment, so that it is especially appropriate for oily skin.

Nettle water

100 ml (6 tbsp) dried nettles
1 litre (3/4 pt) distilled water
1/4 tsp borax
1 pinch sodium benzoate,
    if desired

Nettle water is soothing
and has a considerable
cleansing effect.

Let the nettles simmer in
the water for at least half
an hour, then allow the infusion to stand cold for
twenty-four hours before
straining off the nettles.
Boil about half a decilitre
of water and dissolve the
borax in it, and also the
preservative, if one is to be
used. Add the borax mix-
ture to the nettle water
and pour the resulting mixture into thoroughly
cleaned jars. Keep in a
cool, dry place, such as a
refrigerator.

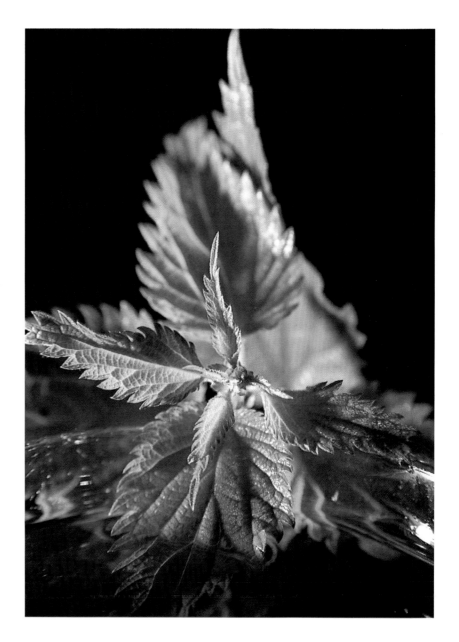

Nettle mask

1 tbsp dried nettles
1 tbsp arrowroot flour
1 tbsp cream
1 tbsp nettlejuice
    (nettle water)
1 teaspoon honey

Nettle masks are excellent for sensitive and irritated complexions.

Mix all the ingredients into a thick, smooth paste. The
dried nettles may well benefit from being left for a while in
a mixture of cream and nettle water. Spread the mask all
over the face, and leave it in place for about twenty
minutes before rinsing with lukewarm water.

Nettle cream

100 ml (6 tbsp) dried nettles
15 g (1/2 oz) white wax
2 tbsp glycerol
15 g (1/2 oz) cocoa butter
4 tbsp almond oil
3 tbsp wheat-germ oil
6 tbsp distilled water
1 pinch sodium benzoate,
   if desired

Nettle cream is excellent for sensitive and nervous complexions.

   Let the nettles simmer in the oil (the almond oil and wheat-germ oil) for at least an hour, then pour the mixture, together with the nettles, into a thoroughly cleaned jar. Leave the jar in a light place for ten days. Separate off the liquid by straining through a thin cloth – muslin or gauze is appropriate. Heat the cocoa butter, the wax and the nettle water in a water-bath, stirring constantly until the mixture is smooth and fine. Meanwhile, heat the distilled water, and if a preservative is to be used, dissolve it in the water. Add the glycerol to the oil mixture, and remove the basin from the water-bath. Then add the hot water, very carefully, while whisking with an electric whisk. Continue whisking until the cream has thickened properly and become

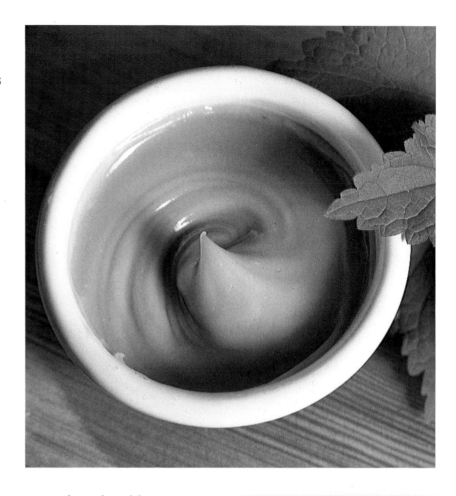

smooth and stable, at which point a small balloon whisk can be used to continue whisking until the cream is really cool. Use a spoon to transfer the cream into a thoroughly cleaned jar, and keep it in a cool, dark place but not in a refrigerator.

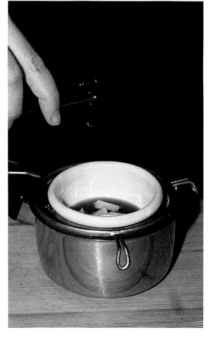

Rose

The rose is one of the oldest beautifying flowers in the world. It has been used for its scent, and for its softening, moisturizing and refreshing qualities. Rose water is astringent, and is often used in creams and lotions. Rose oil is used as a fragrant oil, and one or a few drops are sufficient to add perfume to a whole batch of skin cream.

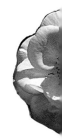

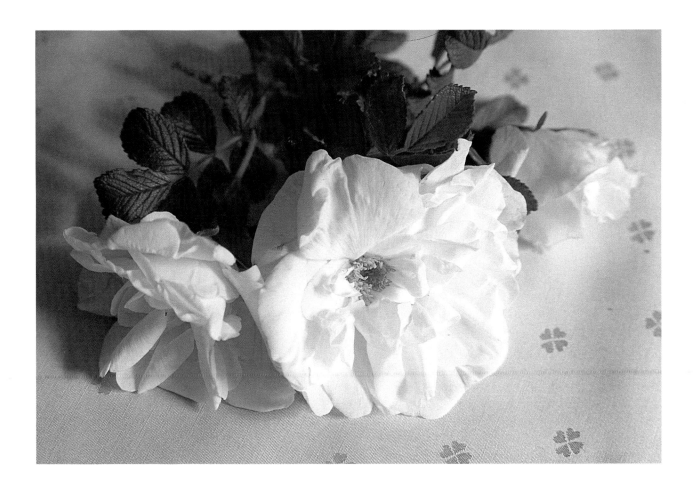

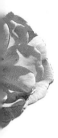

Simple rose water

700 ml (1 1/4 pt) fresh rose
    petals
800 ml (1 3/8 pt) distilled
    water
1 1/2 tsp borax

Use rose water as an astringent face lotion, or as a liquid in creams and lotions. Rose water is suitable for all types of skin.

Rinse the rose petals thoroughly, then chop them or reduce them in a mixer. Boil the water and pour it over the rose petals, which should be in an enamel or stainless-steel vessel. Allow the mixture to cool, then transfer the rose water, petals and all, into a stainless steel saucepan and simmer for a short while; add the borax, and stir. Do not strain, but pour the rose water into a thoroughly cleaned bottle and stand in a light place for a few days. Strain, and transfer the clear rose water into a thoroughly cleaned glass bottle or jar. Keep in a cold place.

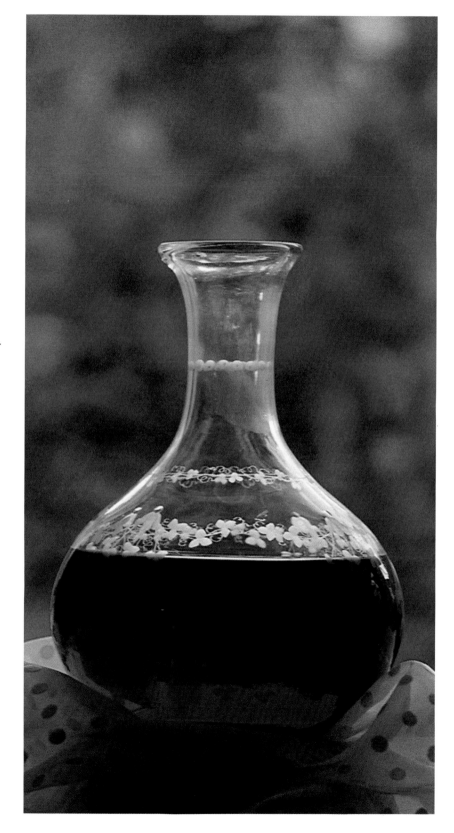

Refreshing face lotion with roses

3 tbsp rose petals
1 tbsp blackcurrant or
    raspberry leaves
1 tbsp sage leaves
1 teaspoon camomile
    flowers (dried)
150 ml (1/4 pt) distilled
    water
50 ml (3 tbsp) apple-cider
    vinegar
200 ml (7 fl oz) simple rose
    water

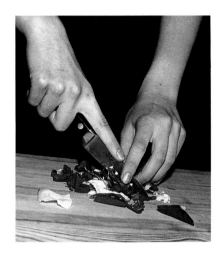

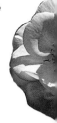

(Left) **Chop the rose petals and the blackcurrant and sage leaves.**

(Below) **Pour boiling distilled water over them.**

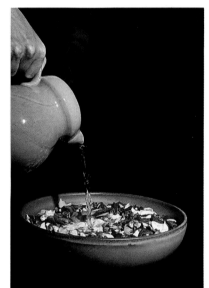

This face lotion refreshes, but is also astringent. It can be used as an after-shave.

Rinse the rose petals, blackcurrant, and sage leaves extremely carefully in hot water, then place all the leaves in a glass jar. Heat the vinegar and water, and pour over the leaves: close immediately with a lid, and let the mixture stand for a week in a refrigerator before straining and adding the rose water. A little borax may be added as a preservative; rose water does contain borax, but a little more may well be needed. Keep the face lotion in a cold, dark place.

Rose mask

200 ml (7 fl oz) fresh rose
    petals
1 tbsp cream
2 tbsp almond oil
50 ml (3 tbsp) oatmeal
    (crushed hulled oats)
a little distilled water,
    if desired

A rose mask livens up tired skin, and even tones and makes the skin smooth.

Rinse the rose petals thoroughly, then chop or reduce in a mixer. Mix the petals with the oatmeal, almond oil and cream; if the mask needs a little more moisture, add distilled water until it forms a smooth and easily workable paste. Apply the rose mask and leave in place for at least half an hour, then rinse away with lukewarm water.

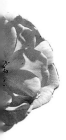

Rose cream 1

30 g (1 1/4 oz) beeswax
215 ml (7 1/2 fl oz) almond oil
1 tbsp glycerol
175 ml (6 fl oz) rose water
1 teaspoon borax
1 pinch sodium benzoate if desired

Rose cream is moisturizing and suitable as a night cream.

Melt the wax and the oil in a water-bath. Meanwhile, heat but do not boil the rose water. Then stir the oil mixture gently until it is clear and smooth, and add the glycerol while stirring all the while. Dissolve the borax and the sodium benzoate, if any, in the hot rose water. Remove the dish from the water-bath, and add the rose water one spoon at a time while whisking vigorously with an electric whisk. Keep whisking until the cream has cooled down almost completely, then continue beating with a small balloon whisk. When the cream is cold, spoon it into a thoroughly cleaned jar, and keep it in a cool, dark place.

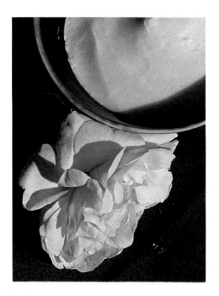

Rose cream 2

10 g (1 tsp) white wax
30 g (3 tsp) cocoa butter
2 tbsp almond oil
2 tbsp avocado oil or
   sesame oil
1 tbsp coconut oil
4 tbsp rose extract (see
   below for proportions)
1 pinch sodium benzoate,
   if desired

Melt the wax, cocoa butter and oils in a water-bath, stirring all the time until the mixture is smooth and clear. Meanwhile, heat the rose extract, and if sodium benzoate is required, dissolve it in the extract. Remove the dish from the water-bath, and add the rose extract slowly and carefully while whisking vigorously with an electric whisk. Keep whisking until the cream has cooled, then continue with a small balloon whisk until the cream has cooled down completely. Spoon it into a thoroughly cleaned jar, and keep in a cool, dark place.

Rose extract for the cream can be made by mixing 4 tbsp fresh rose petals and 100 ml (6 tbsp) distilled water. Rinse the petals thoroughly, then boil the water and pour it over the petals. Allow the infusion to draw for a few hours in a container with a lid, then strain off the petals.

Aloe Vera

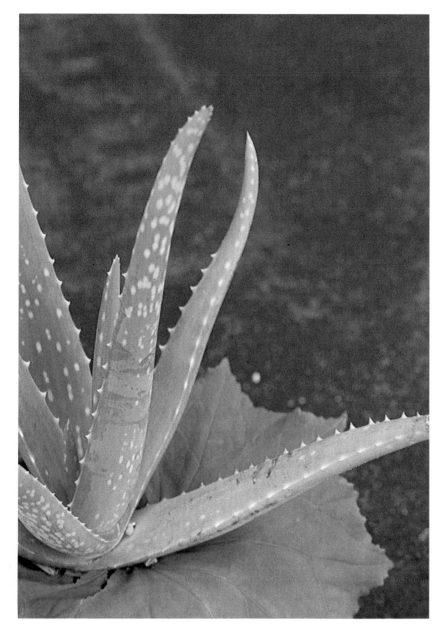

Healing cream

25 g (1 oz) beeswax
6 tbsp coconut oil
5 tbsp almond oil
2 tbsp glycerol
5 tbsp aloe jelly
1 pinch sodium benzoate,
    dissolved in 1 tbsp heated
    distilled water

Melt the beeswax and almond oil in a water-bath. Add the coconut oil (melted coconut butter), and whisk gently with a balloon whisk. Add the glycerol, stir gently and then remove the basin from the water-bath. Use a spoon to add the aloe jelly and continue whisking with an electric whisk, quite vigorously, until the cream has finished cooling. It may not be necessary to use the electric whisk to the bitter end: once it is clear that the cream has assumed a firm and stable consistency, a balloon whisk may be used.

Aloe Vera, or genuine aloe, has long been known as an essential ingredient in creams and lotions. It is primarily the gelatinous substance in the leaves that is used, and pure aloe jelly can be purchased from any well-stocked health food shop. Aloe is an excellent remedy for burnt or irritated skin: it soothes, softens, and is also a very good moisturizer.

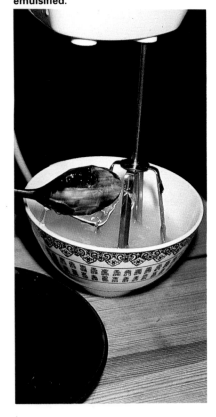

Aloe mask

2 tbsp aloe jelly
4 tbsp finely-ground sweet almonds
2 teaspoons honey
3 tbsp yoghurt

This aloe mask is moisturizing and has a gentle abrasive effect due to the finely-ground sweet almonds.

Mix all the ingredients to form a smooth paste – the best results are obtained with a mixer, but this is not essential. Spread the mask all over the face and neck, and allow it to remain in place for at least twenty minutes before rinsing with lukewarm water.

When the lotion "whitens", it has emulsified.

Moisturizing lotion

25 g (1 oz) cocoa butter
75 ml (4 1/2 tbsp) almond oil
3 tbsp coconut oil
2 tbsp glycerol
75 ml (4 1/2 tbsp) elderflower water
4 tbsp aloe jelly
1 pinch sodium benzoate, if desired

Heat the cocoa butter and oils in a water-bath. When the cocoa butter has melted completely and the mixture is warm but not hot, add the glycerol and beat gently with a balloon whisk. Heat the elderflower water to about the same temperature as the oil mixture. Remove the latter from the water-bath and add very slowly the warm elderflower water, whisking all the time with an electric whisk. When all the elderflower water has been added, continue whisking until the lotion has cooled somewhat, then add the aloe jelly a little at a time and continue whisking at relatively high speed. Keep whisking until the lotion has cooled completely, then pour into a dark-coloured jar and keep in a cool place – not the refrigerator. If you wish to use a preservative (sodium benzoate), dissolve it in the elderflower water – sodium benzoate does not dissolve in oil.

Witch-hazel

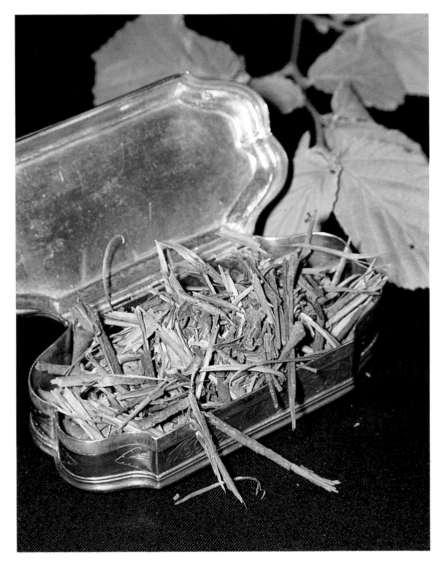

Witch-hazel lotion for oily skin

4 tbsp dried witch-hazel
   bark
600 ml (1 pt) distilled water
20 ml (1 tbsp + 1 tsp) rose
   water
1 tsp borax

This is an astringent and smoothing face lotion which effectively removes excessive oil from the skin. Also good as a shaving lotion.

Boil the distilled water and pour it over the bark. Leave to draw in a sealed container for at least three hours, then strain off the bark and boil the witch-hazel lotion once more, add the borax and the rose water, and remove the saucepan from the heat source immediately. Shake vigorously and pour off the witch-hazel water into a well-cleaned bottle.

Witch-hazel is first and foremost an astringent herb. Either the bark or the leaves are used in creams and face lotions; the bark is stronger. Witch-hazel is also healing, and good for swellings. Since it is primarily a decorative plant, witch-hazel bark may be difficult to obtain. One can knock on the door of someone who grows it and beg a little bark – only a small amount is required – or resort to ready-made witch-hazel water without additives, obtainable from natural cosmetic shops or natural chemists.

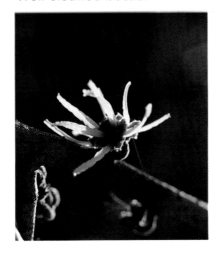

Witch-hazel cream

20 g (3/4 oz) white wax
15 g (1/2 oz) cocoa butter
3 tbsp almond oil
3 tbsp coconut oil
2 tbsp glycerol
1 tsp honey
4 tbsp witch-hazel extract
    (see below for pro-
    portions)
4 tbsp distilled water
1 pinch sodium benzoate,
    if desired

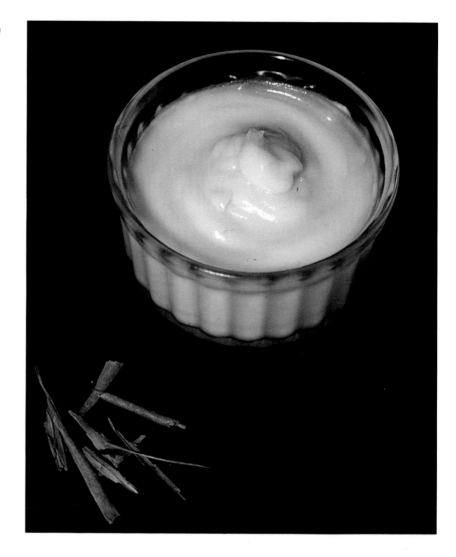

Witch-hazel cream is astringent and very good for mouth sores and oily skin.

Heat the oils, the wax and the cocoa butter in a water-bath, and beat gently with a small balloon whisk until everything has blended and the mixture is clear and smooth. Add the honey while continuing to stir, and then the glycerol. Meanwhile, heat the distilled water mixed with the witch-hazel extract. If a preservative is desired, dissolve it in the liquid and not in the oil mixture. Remove the dish containing the oil mixture from the water-bath and add the hot water very slowly while beating vigorously all the time – an electric whisk gives the best results. Continue whisking until all the water has been added.

When the cream is lukewarm and stable, the electric whisk may be replaced by a small balloon whisk. Continue beating until the cream has cooled down completely. Use a spoon to transfer the cream into a thoroughly cleaned jar, and keep in a cool, dark place, but not in a refrigerator.

Witch-hazel extract is made by mixing 1 tbsp dried witch-hazel bark and 100 ml (6 tbsp) distilled water. Boil the water and pour it over the bark. Allow to draw for three hours, and use the extract for creams and lotions. Some well-stocked health-food shops sell ready-made witch-hazel extract.

Elder

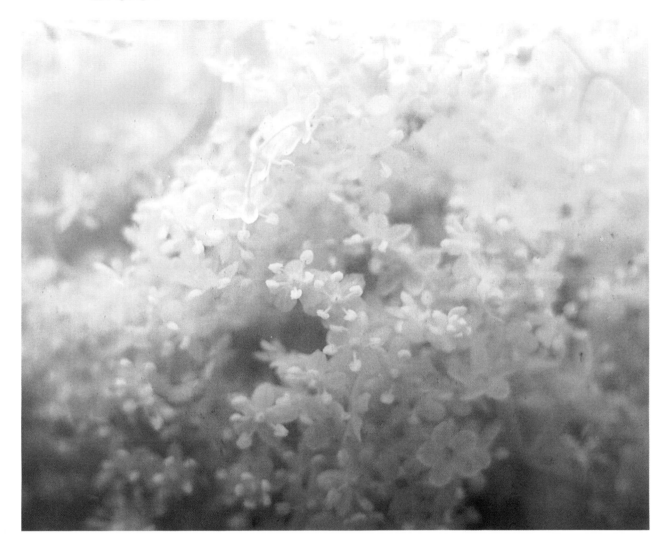

Elder flowers are suitable for all kinds of skin, and in creams and ointments elder tightens the pores and cleanses, besides stimulating circulation of the blood.

Cosmetics are usually made from the blossom of elder bushes, and when you pick elder flowers shortly after midsummer, pay special attention to the colour: there are two kinds of elder, and one of them is poisonous. Only pick the flowers that are pure white in colour: the poisonous strain has a greenish hue.

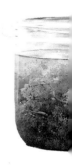

Elder-flower water

8 large clumps of elder
  flowers (10 tbsp dried
  elder flowers)
1 litre (1 3/4 pt) distilled
  water
1/4 tsp borax
1 pinch sodium benzoate,
  if desired

Elder-flower water cleanses
without drying the skin,
and it helps to tighten the
pores. It is also an important ingredient in creams
and lotions.
  Rinse the elder flowers
thoroughly under a cold running tap, then heat the
water and pour it over the
flowers. Leave the infusion
to stand for at least three
hours with a lid in place.
Strain off the flowers, then
add the borax and also the
sodium benzoate dissolved
in a little hot water, if required. After shaking, pour
the elder-flower water into
a well-cleaned jar, and
keep in a refrigerator.

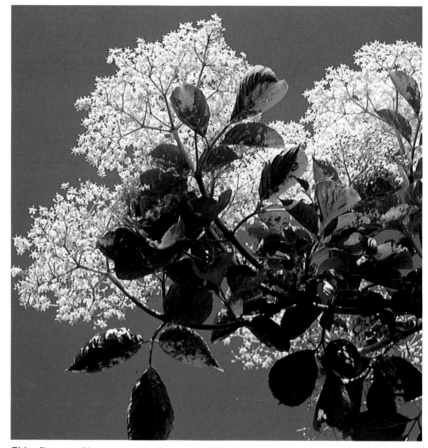

Elder flowers. **Always use the finest, and discard any parts that seem past their prime.**

Eye-freshener with elder flowers

4 tbsp elder flowers
200 ml (7 fl oz) distilled water
2 tbsp glycerol

Rinse the elder flowers under a running hot tap, then boil
the water and pour it over the flowers. Add the glycerol,
and let the mixture stand and brew for a quarter of an hour
before straining off the flowers. Dab two sterile compresses with the elder lotion, then apply the pads to the
eyes. Rest for ten minutes.
  When the compresses are removed, the eyes are clear
and the skin round the eyes smooth and refreshed.

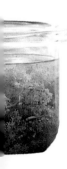

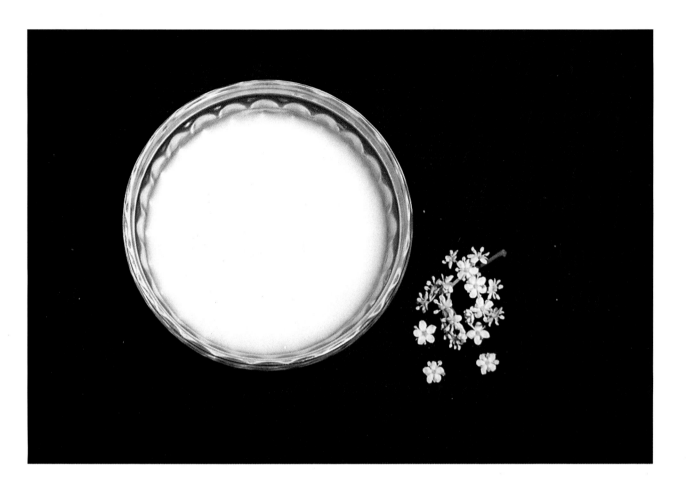

Elder-flower cream

15 g (1/2 oz) white wax
4 tbsp almond oil
2 tbsp coconut oil
2 tbsp thistle oil or sun-
   flower-seed oil
3 tsp glycerol
6 tbsp elder-flower water
1 pinch sodium benzoate,
   if desired

This is an invigorating and stimulating cream for all types of skin.

Melt the wax with the oils in a water-bath, and stir with a small balloon whisk until the wax has melted and the mixture is clear in colour. Heat the elder-flower water: do not boil, but try to keep it about the same temperature as the oil mixture. Then add the glycerol to the oil mixture, and stir. Add the elder-flower water a little at a time, slowly and carefully, stirring quite vigorously all the time with an electric whisk. If sodium bensoate is required, it should be added to the elder-flower water, not to the oil mixture. When all the elder-flower water has been added, keep whisking until it has stabilized. Continue whisking with a small balloon whisk until the cream is completely cool. Spoon the cream into a thoroughly cleaned jar, and keep in a cool, dark place.

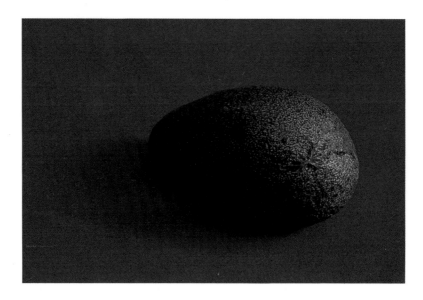

Avocado.

Kelp

Parsley

Cucumber

Olive

Avocado

Carrot

Oats

Cornflower

Wheatgerm

Kelp

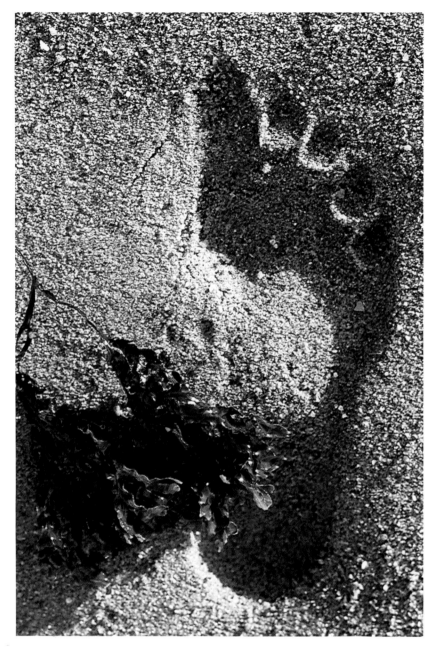

Face mask with kelp

3 tbsp powdered kelp
50 ml (3 tbsp) distilled
 water
2 tbsp rose water
3 tbsp thistle oil or almond
 oil
oatmeal or corn flour

This face mask tones the skin, besides making it smooth and rubbing it clean. It is suitable for all types of skin, but the minerals in the kelp make it particularly appropriate for nervous and easily irritated skin with superficial blood vessels.

 Mix the kelp, distilled water and rose water. Heat the mixture gently, then add the oil and work the ingredients into a smooth paste with the aid of a little oatmeal or corn flour. Apply the face mask, and leave in place for at least half an hour before rinsing away with lukewarm water.

Kelp is in fact the collective name for a large number of brown algae, including such common seaweeds as bladder wrack. It is cleansing, and very good for allergic and nervously blemished skin; it gives the skin moisture and nourishment. Kelp can be found primarily in health-food shops, dried or in powder form.

Parsley

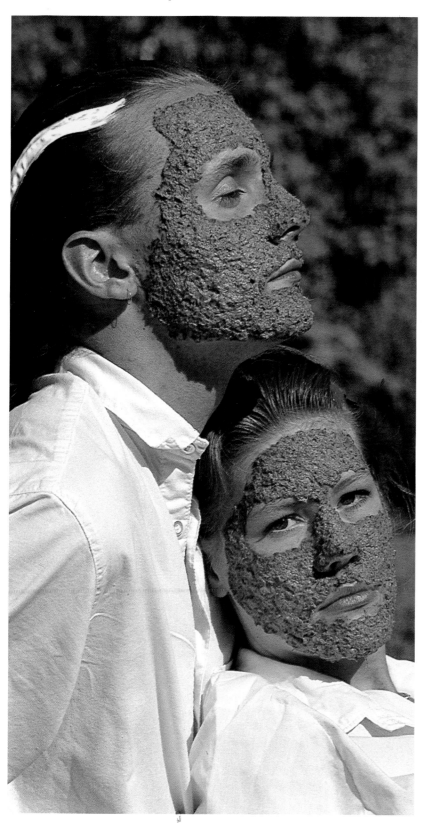

Parsley has a curative effect and is good for oily skin, also for skin which is both oily and troubled with acne.

Parsley mask

100 ml (6 tbsp) finely
  chopped parsley
3 tbsp yoghurt
2 tsp apple-cider vinegar

Parsley masks are good for oily skin: they have a curative effect, and give the skin its correct pH value.
  Mix all the ingredients in a basin, whisking vigorously, then apply the parsley mask and leave in place for at least fifteen minutes.
  Rinse with lukewarm water.

A parsley infusion is good for bathing pimply skin:
  Take 3 tbsp finely chopped parsley and 150 ml (1/4 pt) water. Boil the water and pour it over the parsley, and leave in a container with a lid for at least an hour. Strain, and dab the affected areas with compresses or gauze bandages.

Cucumber

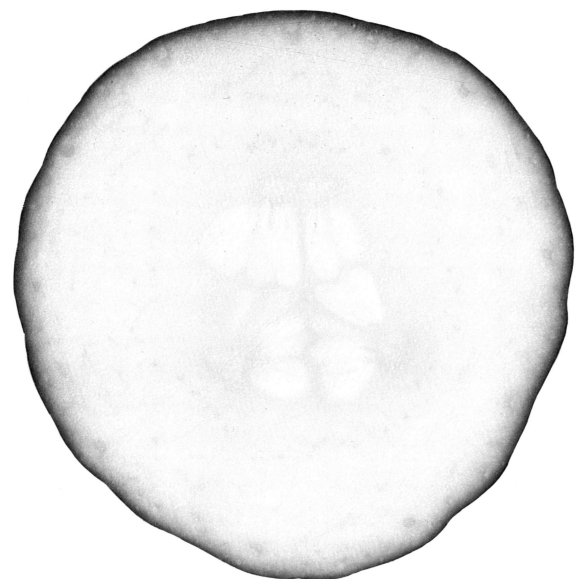

Cucumber juice is refreshing and nourishing. It removes impurities, and also reduces enlarged pores. Cucumber has a tightening effect on pores, and is thus especially good for oily skin. The juice also has a healing effect on burnt skin.

Cucumber water to combat sunburn

1/2 cucumber
1/2 tsp glycerol
1 tbsp elderflower water

Apply liberally to sunburnt skin: it soothes, heals and prevents itching. If made without a preservative (sodium benzoate), cucumber water keeps for only a few days in a refrigerator, so do not be afraid to use lavishly.

Peel and pulp the cucumber, then squeeze out the juice through a thin straining cloth twisted into a spiral. Add the glycerol and the elderflower water. Whisk vigorously and pour off into a thoroughly cleaned jar. Keep in a cold place.

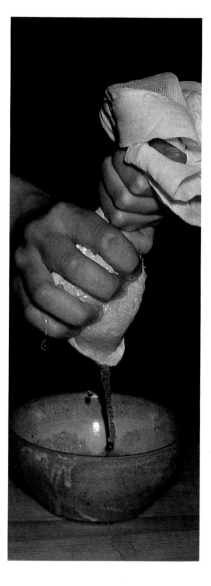

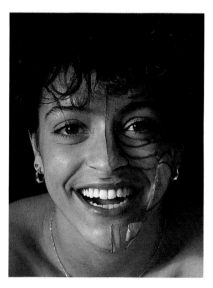

(Left) **The cucumber mask is very astringent and should be used sparingly.**

(Right) **Cucumber lotion is wrung through a fine muslin cloth.**

Cucumber mask

1/2 peeled cucumber
1 egg white
1 tsp lemon juice
1 tsp witch-hazel water
   (can be omitted)
1–2 tsp honey

This cucumber mask should only be used by people with enlarged pores and oily skin, since it has a considerable astringent effect on the pores.

Squeeze the juice out of the cucumber, which is easily done by first grating and then placing the grated pulp in a straining cloth and twisting until all juice has been extracted. Add the lemon juice, witch-hazel, water and honey. Whisk the egg white vigorously, and mix into the cucumber juice. Apply the mask to the face and leave in place for at least a quarter of an hour, or until it has dried out completely, then rinse with lukewarm water.

Face lotion for skin with enlarged pores

4 tbsp cucumber juice
2 tbsp witch-hazel water
150 ml (1/4 pt) elderflower
    water
1/2 tsp borax

This is an astringent face lotion which can also be used as an after-shave.

Mix the cucumber juice, witch-hazel water and elderflower water in a jar with a tight-fitting lid. Shake the jar well, and keep it in a cold place. Then boil a few tablespoons of distilled water and dissolve the borax in it. Pour the liquid into the face lotion and reseal the jar. Keep the face lotion in a cold place.

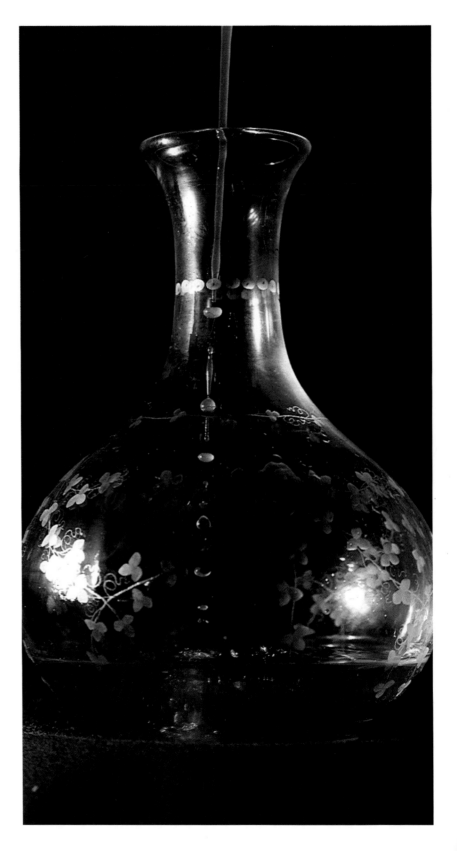

— *Olive* —

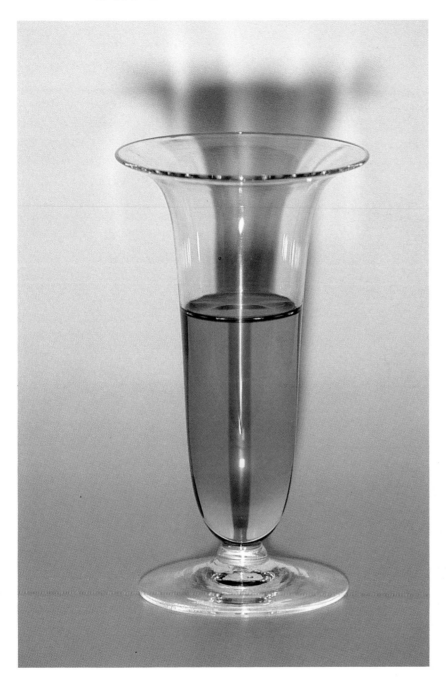

Simple olive ointment for nervous skin

25 g (1 oz) beeswax
150 ml (1/4 pt) olive oil
some drops of rose oil or
    some other fragrant oil, if
    desired

Warm olive oil is good for removing make-up, and is also good for calluses: apply both in the morning and at night for a week, and you will notice a marked improvement.

Heat the olive oil and beeswax in a water-bath, stirring gently until the wax and the oil have fused completely to form a smooth mixture. Remove the dish from the water-bath and add the fragrant oil, if required. Stir until the ointment has cooled completely: an electric whisk is not necessary. Keep the olive ointment in a thoroughly cleaned jar. It is rich in minerals and has a soothing effect.

Olive oil is very fatty and rich in minerals, which means it is good for sore and nervous skin. Always use cold-pressed olive oil, and preferably the green variety, which is most nourishing.

Avocado

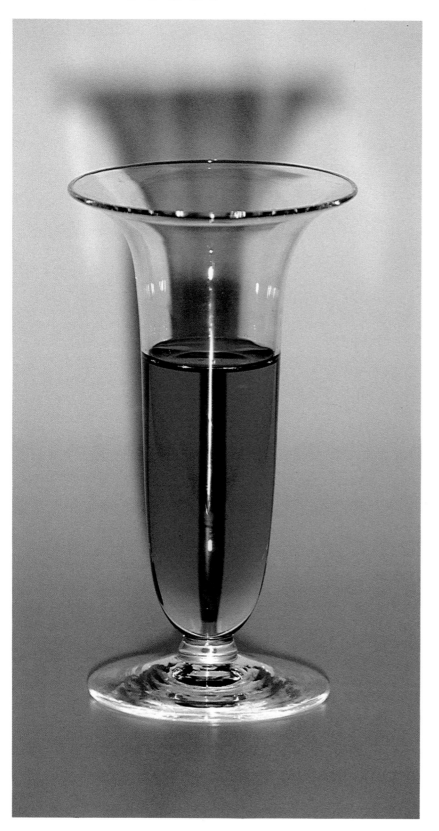

Avocado is especially rich in minerals and vitamins, and hence the oil derived from it is very nourishing. As a result, it is widely used in creams and lotions. Avocado also cleanses, and it gives the skin a bright radiance. It is very good for dry skin.

Cleansing cream with avocado oil

10 g (1 tsp) white wax
1 tbsp lanolin
100 ml (6 tbsp) avocado oil
4 tbsp rose water
1 pinch sodium benzoate,
   if desired

Mix the wax, the oil and the lanolin, then melt the resultant substance in a water-bath, stirring constantly with a small balloon whisk. Keep whisking until the mixture is quite smooth. Meanwhile, heat up the rose water to about the same temperature as the oil mixture – do not allow to boil. If a preservative is required, add it at this point to the rose water. Remove the basin from the water-bath and add the rose water very carefully, whisking vigorously all the time. An electric whisk is best. Keep whisking until the cream has stabilized; you will see when it has "set". The final stages can be done with a balloon whisk. Keep on whisking until the cream is cool, then pour into dark-coloured glass jars and keep in a cool, dry place.

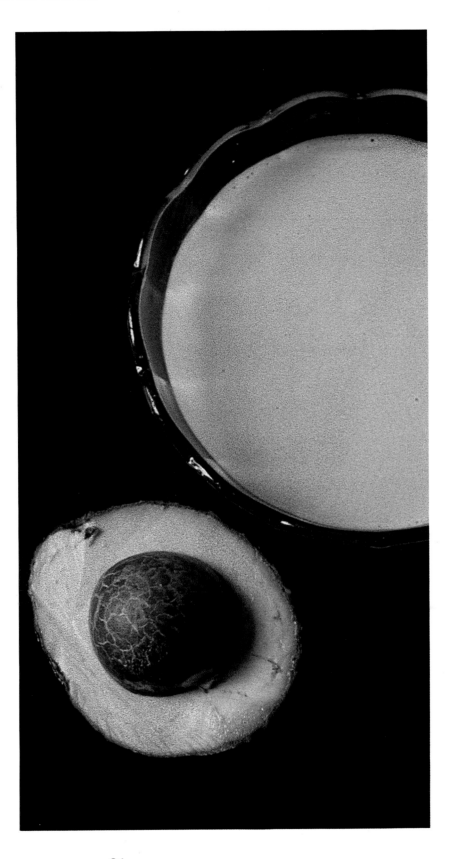

Face mask with avocado

1/2 avocado
2 tbsp almond oil
5 capsules vitamin E
3 tbsp thick cream

Reduce the avocado to a fine pulp, then add the oil. Pierce the vitamin E capsules and squeeze the contents over the mixture. Finally, mix in the cream, preferably after whipping it gently. Stir thoroughly and spread the mask all over the face, with the exception of the eyelids, allowing it to remain in place for some 10 – 15 minutes. Rinse away with lukewarm water.

Light moisturizing cream with avocado

10 g (1 tsp) white wax
10 g (1 tsp)cocoa butter
1 tbsp coconut oil
3 tbsp avocado oil
3 tbsp sesame oil
1 tbsp glycerol
5 tbsp distilled water
1/2 tsp borax
1 pinch sodium benzoate,
   if desired

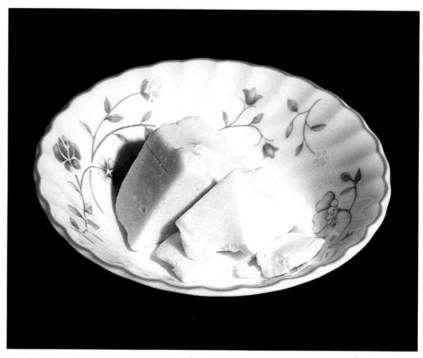

Cocoa butter.

Mix the oils with the water and the cocoa butter, and melt the mixture in a water-bath. When it is quite smooth and clear, it is time to heat up the distilled water: it should not be allowed to boil, but ideally should be kept at about the same temperature as the oil mixture – if the latter gives off steam, it is too hot. Dissolve the borax in the water, and if a preservative is to be added, it should also be dissolved in the heated water. Add the glycerol to the oil mixture, remove it from the water-bath and pour in the hot distilled water, very little at a time, while whisking with an electric whisk. Keep whisking until the cream is smooth and has stabilized, by which time it will have turned rather white in colour. Keep whisking with a balloon whisk until the cream has cooled completely, then use a spoon to transfer it into thoroughly cleaned, dark-coloured jars. It should be stored in a cool, dark place – not a refrigerator, since that would cause the cocoa butter to harden and the cream to separate.

Carrot

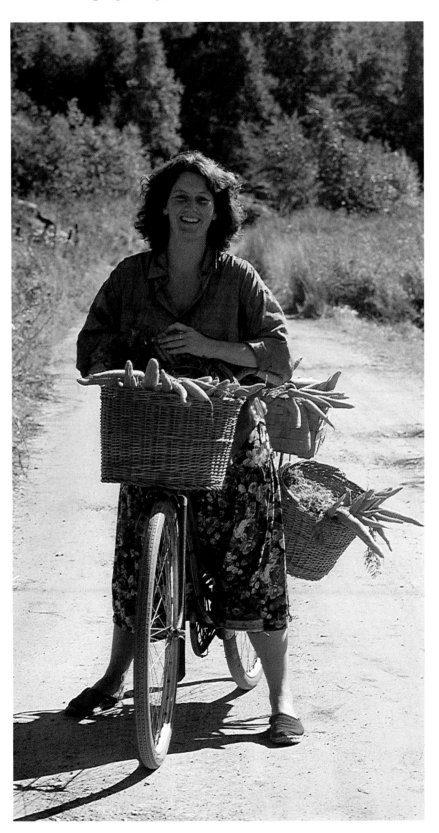

Carrots are rich in vitamin A, and therefore have a certain healing effect on dry skin and chaps. Carotene, the reddish-yellow colouring agent in carrots, is an excellent moisturizer. Carrot oil is good for softening the skin.

Carrot mask

1 carrot
4 tbsp yoghurt
1 tbsp honey
distilled water
oatmeal

This carrot mask is refreshing for the skin. It is moisturizing and nourishing, besides giving the skin an attractive radiance.

Grate the carrot very finely, then mix the grated carrot with the yoghurt and a little distilled water – just a few tbsp to begin with. Heat the carrot mixture in a thick-bottomed saucepan, and allow it to simmer – not boil – for about twenty minutes. Then add the honey and enough oatmeal (crushed hulled oats) to make a workable paste. Apply the face mask and leave it in place for at least fifteen minutes before rinsing with lukewarm water.

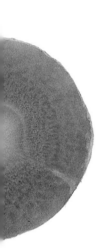

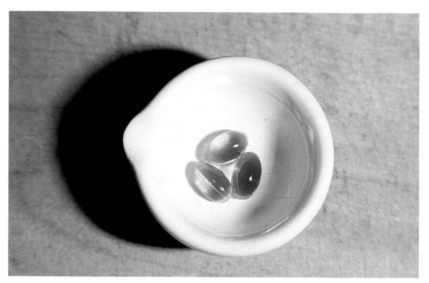

Vitamin E capsules.

Carrot oil for massaging wrinkles

1 large carrot
300 ml (1/2 pt) almond oil
   or sesame oil
2 tbsp honey
6 vitamin E capsules
some drops fragrant oil,
   if desired

Carrot oil is especially good for dry and wrinkled skin.

Peel the carrot and grate it finely with a grater or a mixer. Carefully heat the honey and oil, add the grated carrot, and allow to simmer in a saucepan with a lid for about three hours. The oil must in no circumstances become too hot. Remove the saucepan from the heat, and whisk the oil until it is almost cool. Stick a hole in the vitamin E capsules and squeeze the contents into the carrot oil. Whisk once more, then allow the oil to stand and draw for some hours. Strain away the grated carrot through a cheese cloth, and pour the carrot oil into a thoroughly cleaned bottle. Keep in a cold place.

Carrot cream

10 g (1 tsp) beeswax or
   white wax
1 tbsp lanolin
2 tbsp glycerol
3 tbsp almond oil
3 tbsp thistle oil
1/2 tsp borax
4 tbsp pure pressed carrot
   juice
3 tbsp distilled water
1 pinch sodium benzoate,
   if desired

Melt the wax, lanolin and oils in a water-bath, stirring gently all the time with a small balloon whisk, and when the mixture is smooth and clear, allow it to stand in the water-bath a little longer. Meanwhile, heat the distilled water together with the carrot juice (which must have been sieved and boiled once beforehand), and add borax to the liquid as well as a preservative if so desired. Pour the glycerol into the warm oil mixture and stir once again for some time. Remove the dish from the water-bath, and use a spoon to add slowly the pure carrot juice mixed with the distilled water. Whisk all the time now – an electric whisk is essential in order to obtain perfect results. Keep on whisking until the cream is

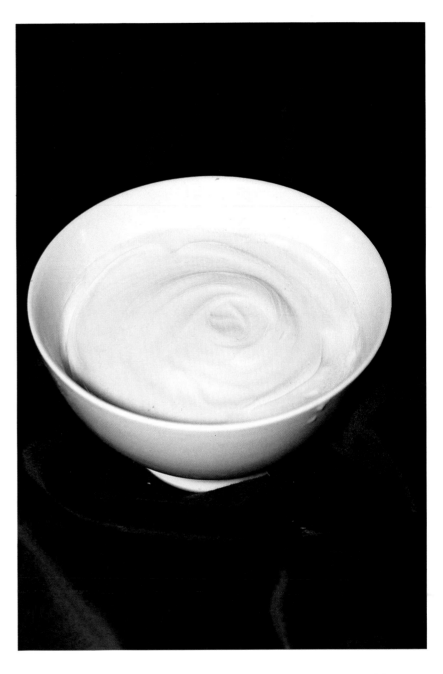

lukewarm, and indeed has almost cooled down altogether, then continue beating with a small balloon whisk until it is quite cold. Add a few drops of fragrant oil if required. Use a spoon to transfer the

cream into a thoroughly cleaned jar, and store in a cool, dry place.

Oats

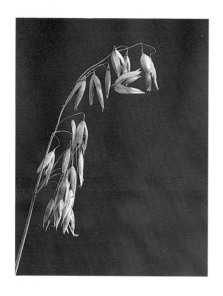

Nourishing mask with oats

200 ml (7 fl oz) crushed
   hulled oats
2 tbsp honey
2 tbsp almond oil
2 tbsp glycerol
rose water or distilled
   water, if desired

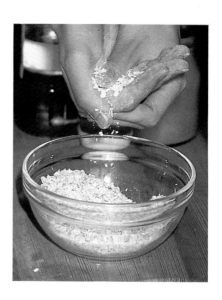

Oats are beneficial, especially for dry skins; oatmeal and oatmeal soap are also soothing for allergic skins. Moreover, oats have an abrasive effect, which makes them most appropriate for use in face masks. Chapped skin becomes soft again after rubbing with oatmeal.

A very useful face mask for all types of skin. Anyone with oily skin can exclude the almond oil.

Mix the oats with the almond oil and enough rose water or distilled water to make a smooth paste. Heat the honey and glycerol in a water-bath, then add to the paste and mix. Apply the mask and leave in place for at least half an hour before rinsing with lukewarm water.

Scrub mask with oats

200 ml (7 fl) oz crushed hulled oats
100 ml (6 tbsp) finely-ground sweet almonds (almond flour)
50 ml (3 tbsp) distilled water

This scrub mask makes the skin smooth and soft.

Soak the almonds in the distilled water, then mix in the oats. If the mixture feels too dry, add a little more water. Heat the mixture until it is a little over body temperature, then apply and leave in place for at least fifteen minutes. Use a face-cloth or terry towel to rub the mask into the face using upward rotary movements. Continue rubbing for about five minutes, then rinse away the mask with lukewarm water and gently work a light moisturizing cream into the skin.

Corn flour

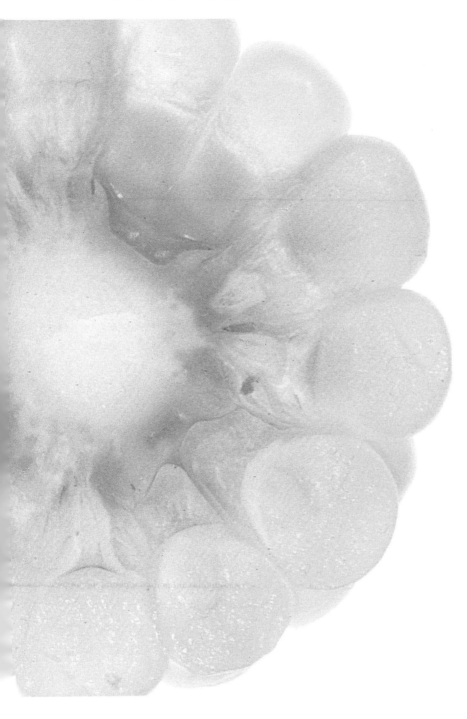

Cleansing face mask with corn flour

150 ml (1/4 pt) corn flour
  (maizena, not polenta)
2 tbsp groundnut oil
2 tsp honey
100 ml (6 tbsp) rose water
distilled water

Mix all the ingredients to form a smooth paste, adding enough distilled water to make the mask easily workable, then heat the mixture carefully. Apply it hot for twenty minutes before rinsing away with lukewarm water.

Corn flour eye-jelly

2 tbsp corn flour (maizena)
elder-flower water

This eye-jelly clarifies the eyes and refreshes the skin around the eyes.
  Heat the corn flour and a little elder-flower water slowly in a thick-bottomed saucepan. When the mixture thickens, add enough elder-flower water to make a workable paste. When cooled, apply it to the eyelids and around the eyes for about fifteen minutes before rinsing away with lukewarm water.

Corn flour softens the skin, is a gentle abrasive and also makes the skin glow; it is especially useful for face masks. It is kind to the skin, and seldom gives rise to allergies.

Wheatgerm

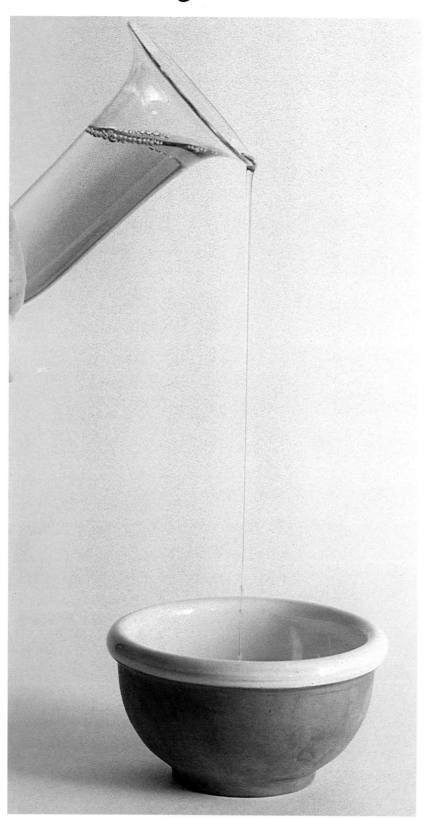

Wheatgerm is very rich in vitamin E, and hence nourishing for the skin. Wheatgerm oil can be used on its own, or as a skin oil in creams or ointments. Both wheatgerm and wheatgerm oil are moisturizers and neutral, and they seldom cause skin allergies.

As wheatgerm oil has a smell all of its own which does not appeal to everybody, it may be appropriate to add a few drops of fragrant oil.

Wheatgerm mask

100 ml (6 tbsp) wheatgerm
2 tbsp wheatgerm oil
2 tsp honey (can be omitted)
2 tbsp yoghurt
50 ml (3 tbsp) distilled water

Wheatgerm cream.

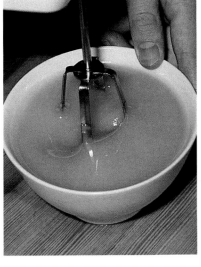

This wheatgerm mask is nourishing and moisturizing. It is neutral, and suitable for all types of skin.

Mix all the ingredients and stir to form a smooth paste, then apply the mask and leave in place for about half an hour. Rinse off with lukewarm water.

Wheatgerm cream

10 g (1 tsp) beeswax or
   white wax
15 g (1/2 oz) cocoa butter
5 tbsp wheatgerm oil
4 tbsp rose water
5 vitamin E capsules
1 1/2 tbsp glycerol
1 pinch sodium benzoate,
   if desired

Body oil for dry skin

150 ml (7 1/2 tbsp) wheatgerm oil
50 ml (3 tbsp) almond oil
50 ml (3 tbsp) chopped
   comfrey leaves (if dried
   leaves are used, 2 1/2 tbsp
   are sufficient)

Wheatgerm.

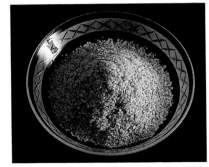

Comfrey is moisturizing and healing, and its qualities are enhanced when mixed with the wheatgerm oil and almond oil. The body oil can be used on the face, and on skin all over the body.

Chop the comfrey leaves finely, or reduce in a mixer, together with the almond oil and wheatgerm oil. (If dried leaves are used, they should be soaked in 3 tbsp distilled water for twenty-four hours before the oil is made.) Let the mixture draw for three days, then strain off the comfrey and squeeze out every drop of oil. A piece of fine cheese-cloth or gauze is usually adequate. Pour the body oil into a thoroughly cleaned bottle, and store in a cold, dark place.

Melt the wax, cocoa butter and oil in a water-bath, stirring until smooth and clear. Heat the rose water. Add the glycerol to the oil mixture and stir. Remove the dish from the water-bath and add the warm rose water, one spoon at a time. Whisk vigorously until the cream has cooled down completely, pierce the vitamin E capsules and squeeze into the cream, stirring all the while.

Keep in a clean jar in a cool, dark place.

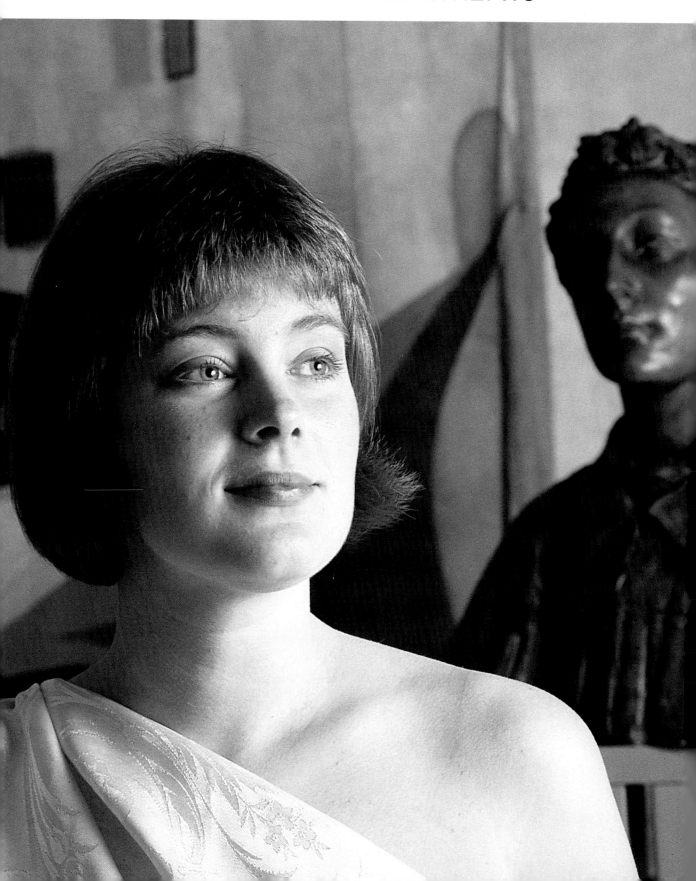

Vitamins A, B and E are the ones used primarily in vitaminizing face masks. Vitamin A has a healing and anti-inflammatory effect, vitamin B counters lined and sagging skin, while vitamin E is moisturizing and helps to smooth skin. How much vitamin the skin can absorb from external sources is impossible to say, and so vitamin cures applied to the skin should always be supplemented with a daily intake of vitamins A, B and E, such as brewer's yeast tablets.

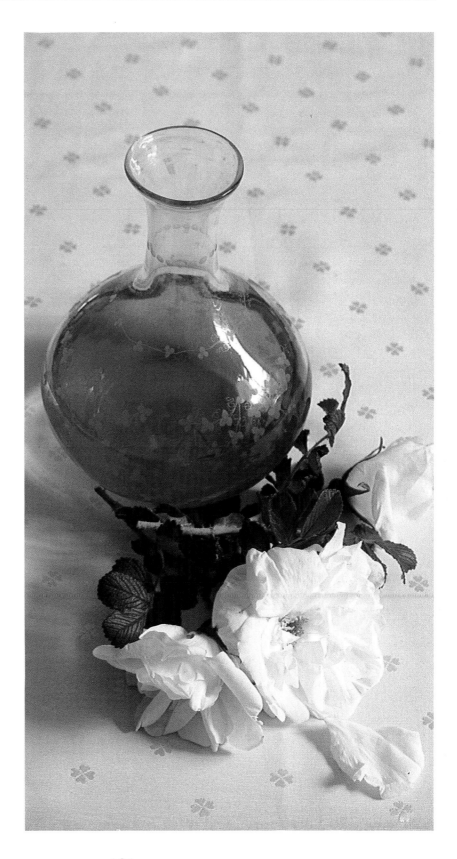

Vitamin B mask 1

1 pkt fresh yeast
1 tsp honey
1 tbsp yoghurt
oatmeal

A marvellous face mask suitable for all types of skin. It cleanses, scrubs and refreshes tired skin.

Stir the yeast and the honey together, and then mix with the yoghurt. Add as much oatmeal (crushed hulled oats) as is necessary to make an easily worked paste. Apply the mask and leave in place for about half an hour, or until it has dried out and starts to crumble. Rinse away with luke-warm water.

Vitamin B mask 2

2 tbsp brewer's yeast
  (powder)
1 tbsp kelp (dried,
  powdered)
2 tbsp corn flour
4 tbsp distilled water

A very nourishing and refreshing mask with a slight ab-rasive effect. The kelp is very rich in minerals, and calms down nervous skin.

Mix all the ingredients in a stainless-steel saucepan or ovenproof dish, adjusting the amount of distilled water as required. Then heat the face mask in a water-bath, and only apply it when it has reached a temperature of about fifty degrees. Leave in place for about twenty minutes, then rinse away with lukewarm water.

Vitamin B mask 3

2 tbsp brewer's yeast
  (powder)
1 tsp honey
2 tbsp wheatgerm oil
2 tbsp almond oil

A cleansing and nourishing oil mask primarily for dry and nervous skin.

Stir all the ingredients together to form a paste, then apply the face mask and leave in place for about fifteen minutes before rinsing away with lukewarm water.

Vitamin B mask 4

1 packet fresh yeast
3 tbsp almond oil
1 tsp honey
2 tsps cream
1 egg white

This mask is very effective for wrinkles, thanks to both vita-mins A and B. The honey softens and cleanses.

Stir together the yeast and the honey, then mix in the oil and cream and stir all the ingredients to form a viscous paste. Whisk the egg white vigorously and fold it into the paste. Apply the mask immediately – it may in fact be necessary to apply it several times – and leave in place for about half an hour before rinsing off with lukewarm water.

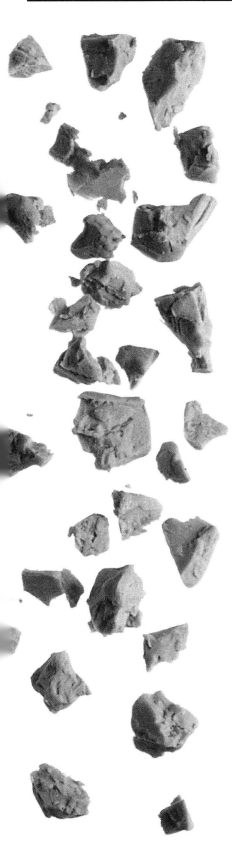

Vitamin E mask 1

6 vitamin E capsules
2 tsp glycerol
3 tbsp distilled water
1 tsp honey
arrowroot flour

A thoroughly effective humectant (moistening) face mask for all types of skin.

Pierce the capsules and squeeze out the contents, being careful to ensure there is nothing left inside. Mix the glycerol, water and honey in a thick-bottomed stainless-steel saucepan, and heat the mixture gently before pouring it over the vitamin E. Add as much arrowroot flour as is necessary to obtain a smooth, workable paste. Apply the face mask and leave in place for at least twenty minutes; if necessary, keep adding new layers as the mask dries out. Rinse away with lukewarm water, being careful not to rub, and allow the skin to dry of its own accord. Wait for a while before applying a light moisturizing cream.

Fresh yeast.

Lecithin granules.

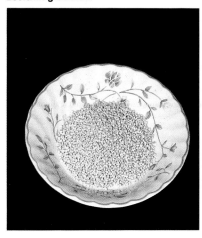

Vitamin E mask 2

3 tbsp wheatgerm oil
2 tbsp cream
2 tbsp granulated lecithin
distilled water

This face mask is packed with vitamin E, and is very good for wrinkles round the eyes.

Mix the oil, cream and granules, then heat the mixture in a water-bath and stir until the granulated lecithin has dissolved completely. If necessary, add a little distilled water. Apply the face mask and leave in place for about half an hour before rinsing away with lukewarm water.

103

Vitamin E mask 3

2 tbsp granulated lecithin
2 tbsp rose water
2 tsp apple-cider vinegar
3 tbsp wheatgerm oil
100 ml (6 tbsp) finely
  ground sweet almonds

A nourishing and humectant face mask suitable for all types of skin. The almonds give it a gentle abrasive effect.

Mix all the ingredients in a thick-bottomed stainless-steel saucepan, or in an ovenproof dish, then heat the mixture gently. Use a water-bath for the dish. Apply the face mask and leave in place for about twenty minutes before rinsing away with lukewarm water.

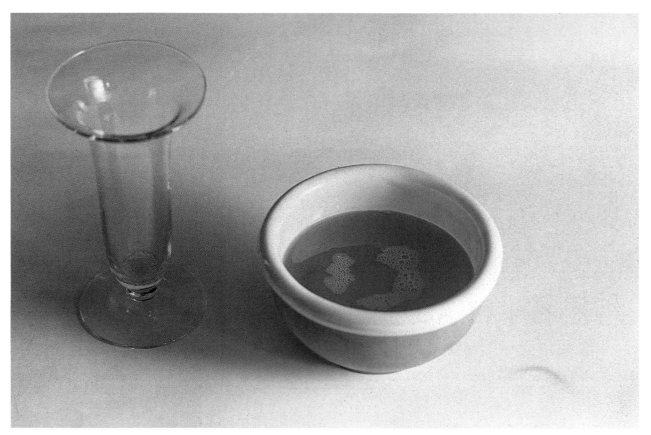

Wheatgerm oil.

Vitamin E mask 4

2 tbsp wheatgerm oil
4 tbsp yoghurt
3 tbsp wheatgerm
2 tbsp oatmeal (crushed
  hulled oats)

A vitamin E mask suitable for all types of skin.

Mix the ingredients in an ovenproof dish and heat the mixture gently in a water-bath. Apply the face mask while it is warm, and leave it in place for about half an hour before rinsing off with lukewarm water.

Vitamin A mask 1

6 vitamin A capsules
2 tbsp avocado oil
1 tbsp rose water
3 tbsp oatmeal
distilled water

A lightly moisturizing and abrasive mask with nourishment from both the capsules and the avocado oil, which is very rich in minerals.

Pierce the capsules and squeeze out the contents, then add the oil, rose water, oatmeal (crushed hulled oats) and a little distilled water. Do not use too much water all at once, or the mask may not be stiff enough. Mix the ingredients thoroughly, and the face mask is ready to apply when the paste is easily workable. Leave it in place for about twenty minutes before rinsing off with lukewarm water.

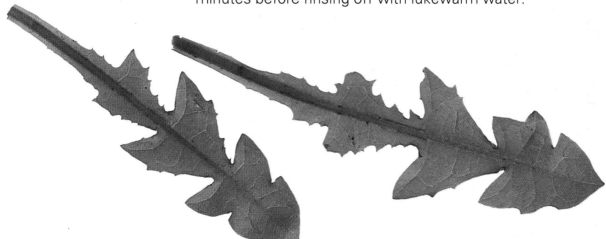

Vitamin A mask 2

3 tbsp crushed dandelion
  leaves
3 tbsp sesame oil
2 tbsp cream
2 tbsp corn flour

This is a cleansing and refreshing face mask with a slight abrasive effect.

Rinse the dandelion leaves very thoroughly, "crush" them or reduce them in a mixer, then mix them with the other ingredients. Apply the face mask and leave in place for about fifteen minutes. Rinse well with lukewarm water, being careful not to rub the skin.

Vitamin A mask 3

1 medium-sized carrot
5 tbsp almond oil
1 tbsp distilled water
2 – 3 tbsp oatmeal
  (crushed hulled oats)

An invigorating mask with a nourishing and moisturizing effect. The oatmeal scrubs and cleanses in depth.

Finely grate the carrot and mix with the oil. Heat the mixture gently, then leave to draw in a saucepan with a lid for two days. Strain the carrot oil through a cheese-cloth, and mix it with the water and oatmeal. Apply the face mask thinly, and leave for fifteen minutes at most before rinsing away with lukewarm water.

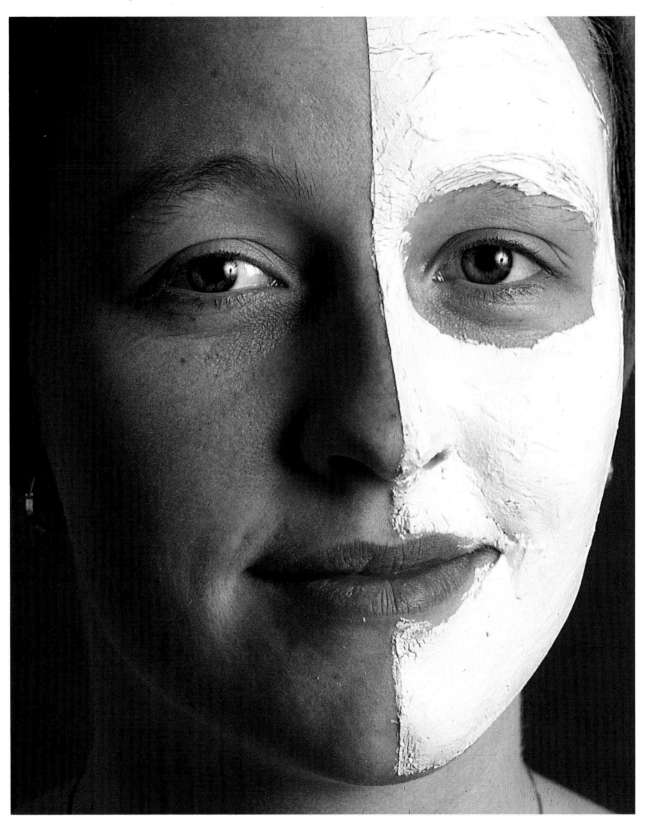

In cases of oily and grubby skin, deep-seated dirt and deep-seated excessive greasiness, a suitable treatment is a clay mask based on either kaolin or Fuller's Earth. Clay masks are very astringent, and should therefore be used only sparingly on dry and nervous skin. Both kaolin and Fuller's Earth are sold in powder form by chemists.

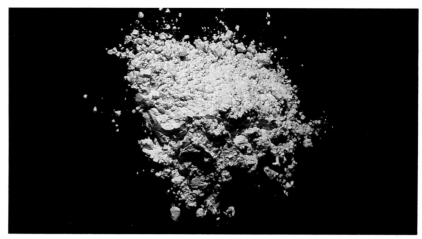

Kaolin.

Clay mask for acne

2 tbsp kaolin
1 tbsp dried yarrow
2 tbsp yoghurt
1/2 – 1 teaspoon distilled water

This is a cleansing and very astringent face mask suitable only for oily and grimy skin.

Mix all the ingredients to form a thick paste. Be careful with the water, and use a little at a time so as to keep control of the consistency: the mask must not be runny. Apply the mask evenly all over the face, but avoiding the area around the eyes, and leave in place for ten minutes. Rinse away with lukewarm water: avoid rubbing, but let the mask simply wash away.

Simple clay mask

2 tbsp kaolin
1 tbsp well-whisked egg white
1 tbsp cucumber juice
2 tsp yoghurt

A simple and easily prepared face mask. It cleanses and reduces large pores.

Mix all the ingredients to form a smooth paste and apply it, avoiding the area around the eyes. Leave in place for ten minutes before rinsing away with lukewarm water.

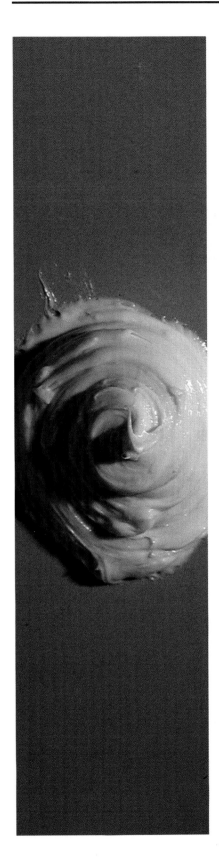

Cleansing clay mask

5 g (1/2 tsp) beeswax
2 tbsp lanolin
5 tbsp rose water (heated)
100 g (3 1/2 oz) kaolin

This clay mask cleanses in depth. The lanolin has a softening and astringent effect.

Melt the wax and the lanolin in a water-bath, and add the heated rose water a little at a time while whisking vigorously – preferably with an electric whisk. Add the kaolin and stir until the paste is smooth and even. Apply the face mask, avoiding the area around the eyes. Leave in place for ten minutes before rinsing away with lukewarm water.

(Left) **Lanolin.**

Clay mask with kelp

2 tbsp kaolin
1 tbsp kelp (dried)
4 tbsp distilled water
1 tbsp honey

A refreshing and cleansing face mask which can also be used on normal skin.

Add the water to the kelp, and allow it to stand and swell for a few hours; the liquid will be rather treacly and sticky. Add the clay and honey to the kelp, and stir: it may be necessary to add a few more drops of water, a little at a time. When the paste is smooth and even, apply the face mask but avoid the area around the eyes. Leave the mask in place for about ten minutes, then rinse it away with lukewarm water.

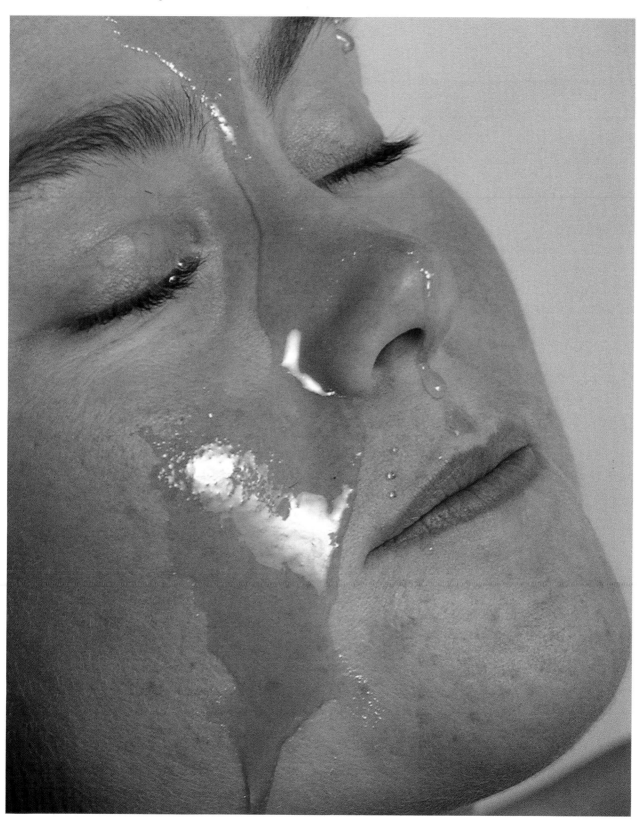

Honey has always been used for rejuvenating purposes. It can be used with all types of skin, but is especially effective with dry and chapped skin. It cleanses and heals, and easily removes dead skin cells besides being a moisturizer. When you use honey in face masks and creams, you should ensure that it is unboiled, since it is more effective then.

Good health-food shops should stock some brands of honey which have not been boiled during processing. It is worth checking the labels on the jars for this information.

Cleansing massage lotion for oily skin

3 tbsp honey
2 tsp lemon juice
1/2 whisked egg white
2 tsp apple-cider vinegar

This massage stimulates the blood circulation and cleanses in depth. The lotion is astringent and has a smoothing effect.

Mix all the ingredients. Cleanse the face thoroughly and work in the lotion, starting with the throat. Continue with rotary motions up to the forehead, then rinse with lukewarm water.

Cleansing massage lotion for dry skin

3 tbsp honey
2 tbsp almond oil
2 tbsp apple-cider vinegar

A softening and cleansing massage. The apple-cider vinegar normalizes the pH value of the skin.

Mix all the ingredients to form a smooth lotion, then proceed as in the previous recipe before rinsing with lukewarm water.

Blackhead treatment

4 tbsp honey
1 1/2 tbsp wheat germ
some drops apple-cider vinegar

Heat all the ingredients in a water-bath. When the honey has become tacky and the mixture has just begun to steam, remove the dish from the water-bath and start massaging the areas affected by blackheads with rotary motions. Apply a thin layer of the honey mixture, and leave in place for about ten minutes before rinsing with lukewarm water. After this treatment, it should be easy to remove the blackheads.

Honey and olive oil mask

3 tbsp honey
3 tbsp olive oil
gauze

This treatment is excellent for tired and wrinkled skin. Both the honey and the olive oil are rich in minerals, and in combination they supply the skin liberally with moisture and nourishment.

Mix the honey and the olive oil in an enamel saucepan, and heat the mixture to form a smooth, viscous paste. Cut the gauze into pieces three decimetres long and dip them into the oil mixture, then apply them to the skin at the hottest tolerable temperature until the whole face is covered. Cold compresses can be applied to the eyelids in order to protect the eyes. Leave the gauze in place for at least twenty minutes, then rinse carefully with lukewarm water, followed if desired by a little rose water.

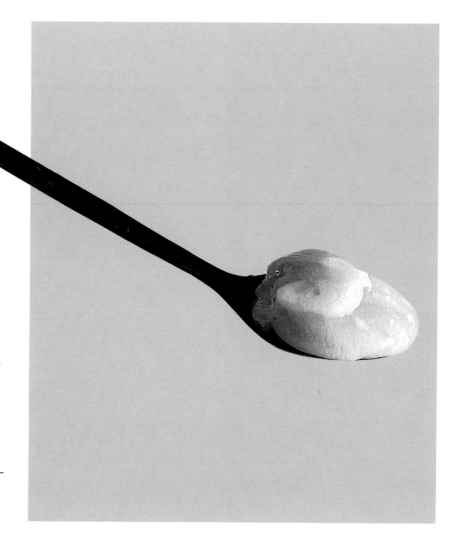

Anti-wrinkle mask

4 tbsp honey
2 tbsp thick cream

A really refreshing treatment which has both a cleansing and a smoothing effect.

Heat the honey and cream in a water-bath. As soon as the mixture begins to steam, remove the dish from the water-bath. Apply the face mask at as high a temperature as is tolerable, and if necessary keep adding layers. Leave the mask in place for at least fifteen minutes, then massage the face thoroughly with upward rotary movements. Rinse with lukewarm water and allow the face to dry of its own accord.

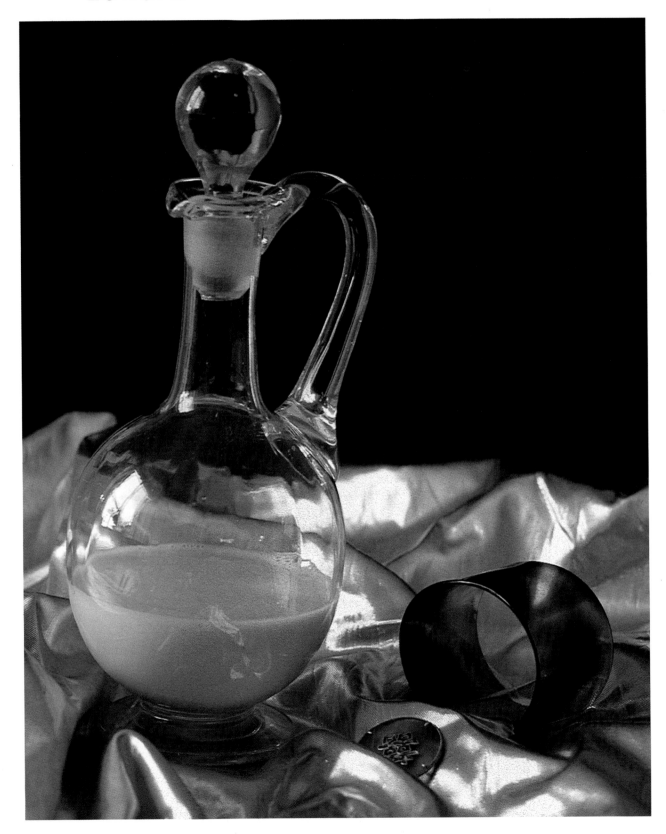

These days, when people take a shower once and perhaps even twice a day, if there is one thing the skin needs, it is moisture. The easiest way to provide moisture is by using a body lotion after the shower. You can make the most marvellous lotions yourself, and after a while, once you have learnt the basic technique and you feel confident about how to make your own lotions, you can start experimenting – substituting a particular oil for something else, or some herbal extract for a raw juice, perhaps. Eventually, you will find a lotion which suits your skin perfectly.

Mainly water

As distinct from creams, lotions consist mainly of water or liquid. A lotion is an emulsion of the "oil-in-water" type, and in order to make the oil and water mix to form a homogeneous solution, some form of emulsifier has to be added. Otherwise, the result is rather like a dressing – vinegar at the bottom and oil at the top. Put at its

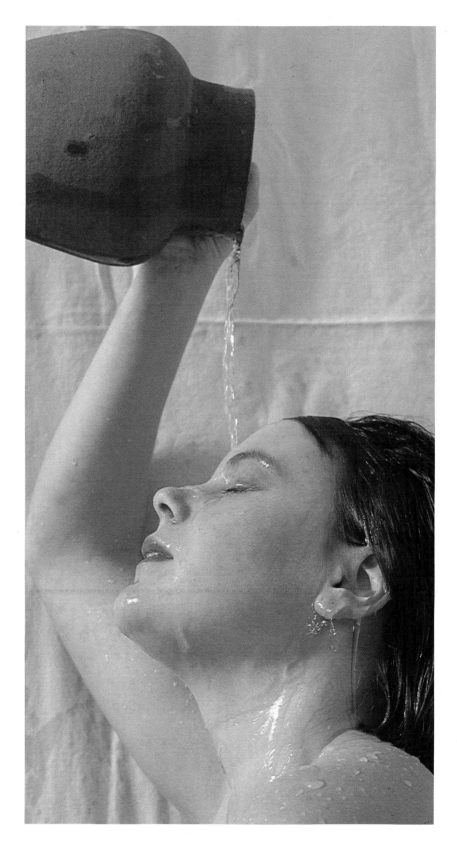

simplest, an emulsifier helps two normally incompatible substances to blend and form a stable solution.

Emulsifiers

I have tried various emulsifiers and found from experience that the best emulsifier as far as lotions are concerned is lecithin. Cholesterol is certainly a conceivable alternative, but it is very expensive, whereas lecithin is quite reasonable in price. It is essential that you should use absolutely pure granulated lecithin, with no trace of added vitamins or any other substance. All well-stocked health-food shops keep granulated lecithin.

When you make a lotion, it is important that you should use an electric whisk, and equally vital that you should continue whisking until the lotion has cooled down completely.

The emulsifying process

Oils have differing emulsifying properties, but you will see in the case of a lotion that when it starts to emulsify, it turns white, its colour becomes richer in quality, and it changes its consistency somewhat.

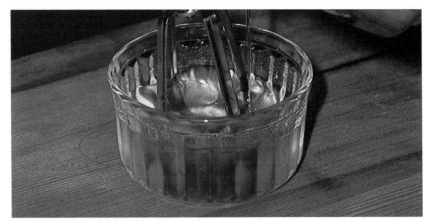

1. Both liquid and oil must have the same temperature.

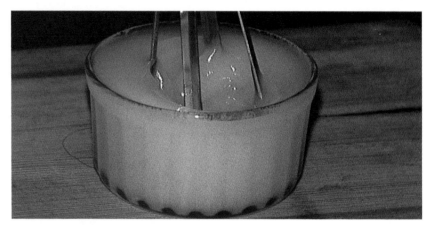

2. When the mixture whitens, it has emulsified.

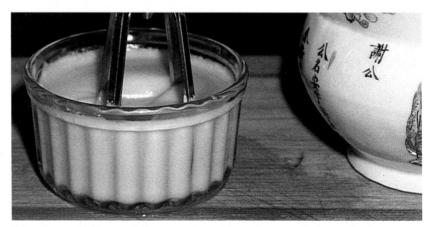

3. Continue whisking until the cream is cool. The photograph shows clearly how smooth the resulting cream is.

When this starts happening, it is essential that you should continue whisking until the lotion has cooled down completely. This cooling process should not take place too quickly, and when it is completed, you must store the lotion in a cool, dark place. If desired, you may add a preservative – sodium benzoate – and a little borax to kill off bacteria.

First the lecithin

Always start by dissolving the lecithin in the oil: this takes some time, and it helps to crush the granules and to stir with a small balloon whisk or a fork. Note – and this is very important – that if the recipe includes wheatgerm oil, either on its own or in combination with some other oil, you should not dissolve the lecithin in the wheatgerm oil, but in the other oil, assuming this is a compound recipe. If the recipe involves wheatgerm oil only, first dissolve the lecithin in a little almond, thistle or sunflowerseed oil and only then mix the solution with the wheatgerm oil. For some reason or other, lecithin does not dissolve in wheatgerm oil but just forms sticky lumps which cling to the whisk.

As in the case of creams, fragrant oils should be used sparingly. Choose modest, gentle fragrances which make their presence felt subtly, rather than ones which overwhelm the senses.

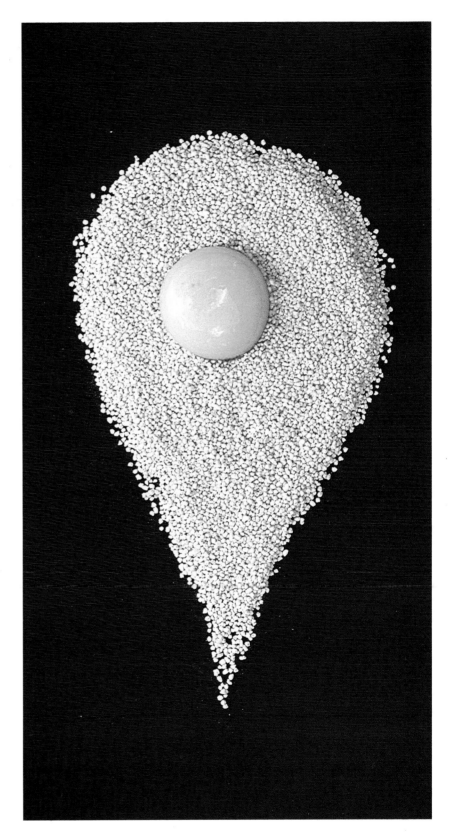

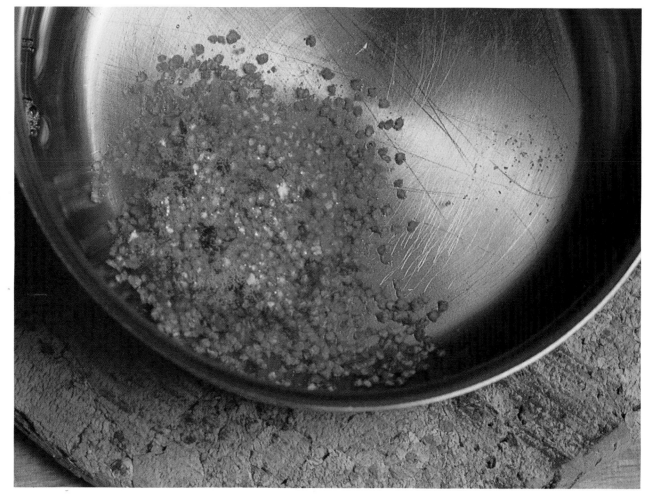

Remove any lecithin granules that do not melt easily.

Tips

If the lecithin granules do not dissolve completely, simply remove the stubborn ones, provided they are not too many – the result is usually satisfactory even so.

Instead of distilled water, you could use carrot juice, strawberry juice, elderflower water, orange-blossom water, nettle water, or similar liquids.

Make sure raw juices are boiled and strained, and that they do not contain particles which could give rise to mould. If desired, add a little borax, which kills off bacteria.

The water or liquid you add to the oil mixture must be hot, and roughly similar in temperature to the oil mixture itself. The liquid should be added a little at a time, while whisking vigorously with an electric whisk. Adding a cold liquid could well disrupt the emulsification process.

Following these instructions is the easiest way of achieving the best results.

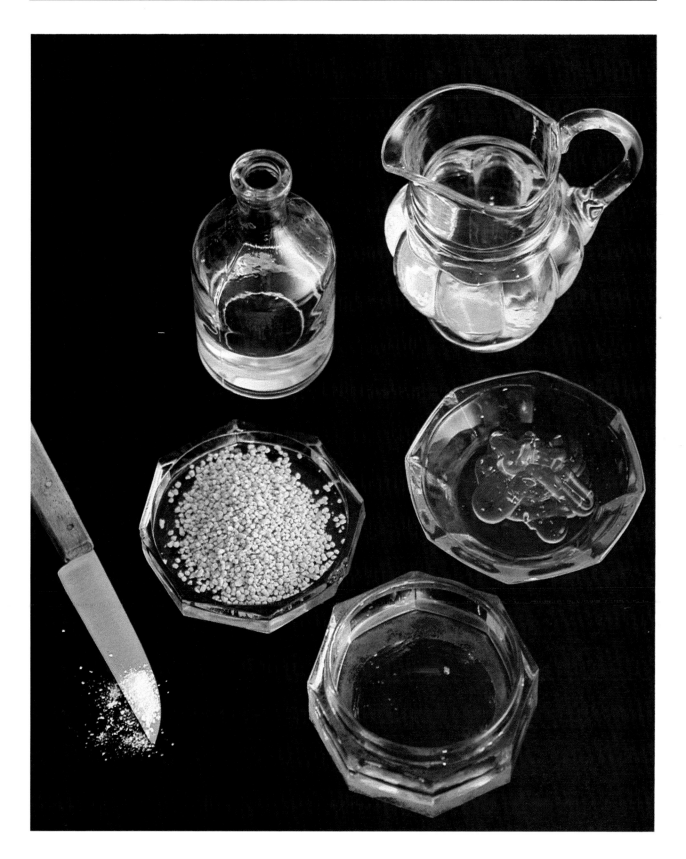

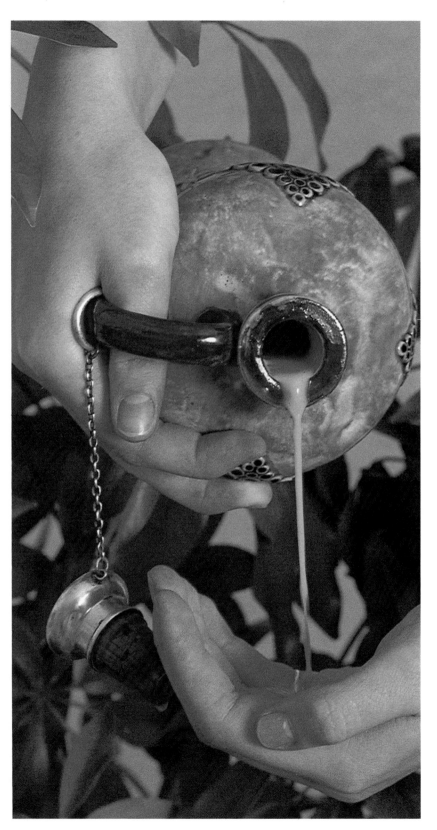

Moisturizing lotion with avocado

2 1/2 tbsp avocado oil
1 tbsp granulated lecithin
1/2 tbsp wheatgerm oil
3 1/2 tbsp glycerol
5 tbsp distilled water
3 tbsp aloe jelly
sodium benzoate,
  if desired

Dissolve the granulated lecithin in the avocado oil, being careful to ensure that it dissolves completely, then add the wheatgerm oil. Use a water-bath as usual, and make sure the mixture is really hot before adding the glycerol. Stir with a small balloon whisk, and meanwhile, heat the distilled water in a sauce-pan and add the sodium benzoate if desired. Remove the dish from the water-bath and add the water to the oil mixture a little at a time, whisking vigorously all the while with an electric whisk. Add the aloe jelly after a short time, and continue whisking until the lotion has cooled down completely. Store it in a dark-coloured bottle, and keep in a cool, dark place.

Body lotion

1 1/2 tbsp thistle oil
1 tbsp granulated lecithin
3 tbsp glycerol
5 tbsp distilled water
fragrant oil and sodium
    benzoate (1 pinch), if
    desired

Dissolve the lecithin and
thistle oil in a water-bath,
and when the lecithin has
dissolved completely, add
the glycerol. Stir with a balloon whisk, then slowly
add hot distilled water. If a
preservative (sodium ben-
zoate) is desired, it should
be dissolved in the hot
water. Remove the dish
from the water-bath and
whisk with an electric
whisk until the lotion has
cooled down completely.
The fragrant oil should be
added last. Store the lotion
in a dark-coloured bottle,
and shake before use.
Keep in a cool, dark place.

Fragrant oil from lily of the valley.

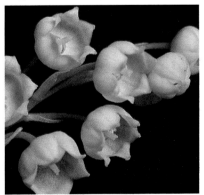

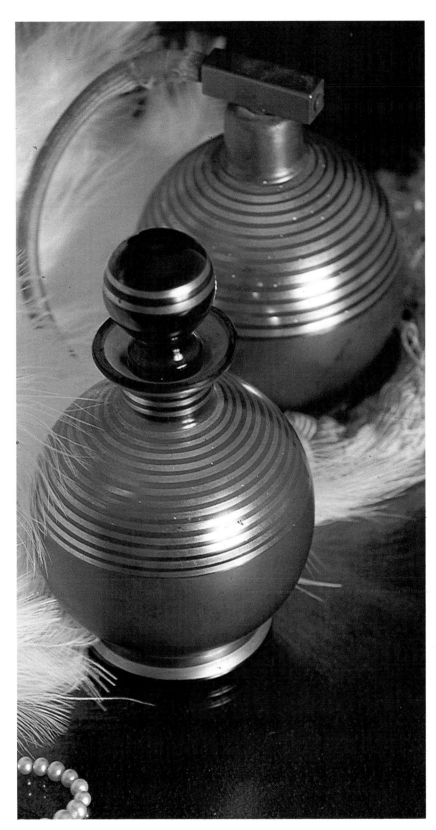

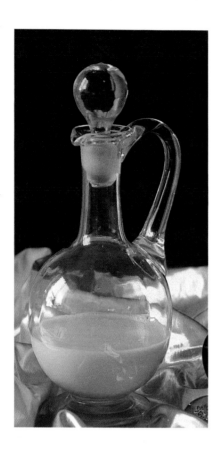

Vitamin E shock for aged skin and wrinkle massage

2 tbsp wheatgerm oil
10 vitamin E capsules
1 tbsp lecithin
1/2 – 1 tbsp thistle or almond oil
3 1/2 tbsp glycerol
7 tbsp distilled water
sodium benzoate, if desired

Thistle oil.

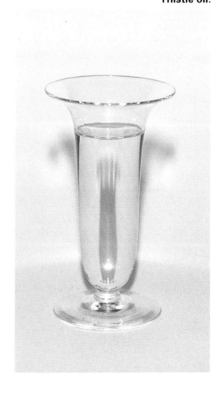

Prepare a water-bath and squeeze out the contents of the vitamin E capsules into a small dish, piercing with a needle if necessary. Add the wheatgerm oil and heat the mixture in the water-bath to about 70 degrees. Dissolve the lecithin in the thistle or almond oil, and when the granules have dissolved completely, pour the mixture into the wheatgerm oil mixture. The lecithin and thistle or almond oil should also be blended in a water-bath. Stir with a balloon whisk. Meanwhile, heat the distilled water, and add the sodium benzoate if desired. Add the glycerol to the oil mixture, and stir. Add the hot water a little at a time, whisking all the while with an electric whisk. Remove the dish from the water-bath, and keep whisking until the lotion has cooled down completely. Add the fragrant oil, if desired.

This lotion is inclined to be a little viscous, and should therefore be stored in a jar rather than a bottle. Use a dark-coloured jar, and keep it in a cool, dark place.

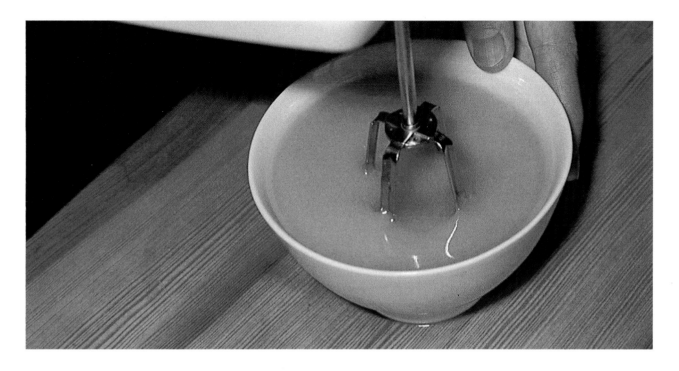

Moisturizing lotion with peach

2 tbsp almond oil
1 tbsp sesame oil
1 tbsp granulated lecithin
10 g (1 tsp) cocoa butter
3 tbsp glycerol
5 tbsp pure peach juice
2 tbsp distilled water
sodium benzoate, if desired
fragrant oil (optional)

Mix the almond oil and sesame oil in a dish, then place the mixture in a water-bath. Dissolve the lecithin completely in the mixture, and add the cocoa butter, beating gently with a small balloon whisk until it has also dissolved completely. Meanwhile, heat the pure peach juice (which should be strained) and the distilled water in a saucepan, and add the sodium benzoate if a preservative is required. Add the glycerol to the oil mixture, and stir. Remove the dish from the water-bath and slowly add the peach juice, beating with an electric whisk. Keep beating until the lotion has cooled down completely, then add the fragrant oil, if desired. Store the lotion in a dark-coloured bottle in a cool, dark place.

Cocoa butter is pressed from the cocoa bean.

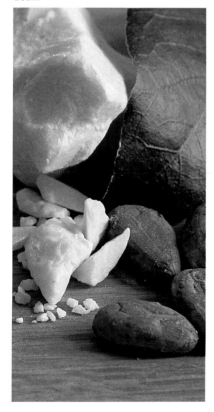

Body lotion

1 1/2 tbsp thistle or almond
   oil
1/2 tbsp avocado oil
1/2 tbsp wheatgerm oil
1 1/4 tbsp granulated
   lecithin
2 tbsp glycerol
7 tbsp distilled water
sodium benzoate, if desired
1 tbsp aloe jelly
fragrant oil (optional)

Heat the thistle or almond
oil and the avocado oil in a
dish, using a water-bath,
then dissolve the granu-
lated lecithin in the oil mixture. Add the wheatgerm
oil and the glycerol, whisking all the time with a small
balloon whisk. Remove the
dish from the water-bath
and slowly add the hot
water, which should con-
tain the sodium benzoate if
any preservative is to be
used. Whisk with an elec-
tric whisk, and add the aloe
jelly after a short while
when the lotion has cooled
down somewhat. Keep
whisking until it has cooled
completely. If a fragrant oil
is desired, it should be
added last of all. Pour the
lotion into a dark-coloured
bottle, and keep in a cool,
dark place.

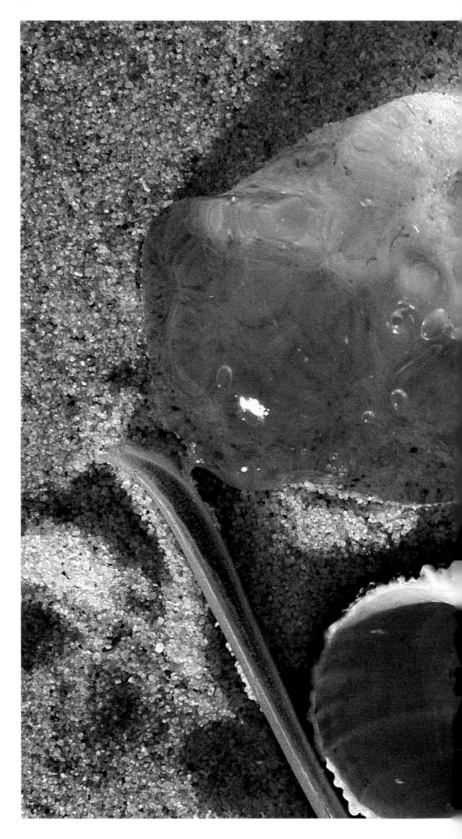

Aloe jelly.

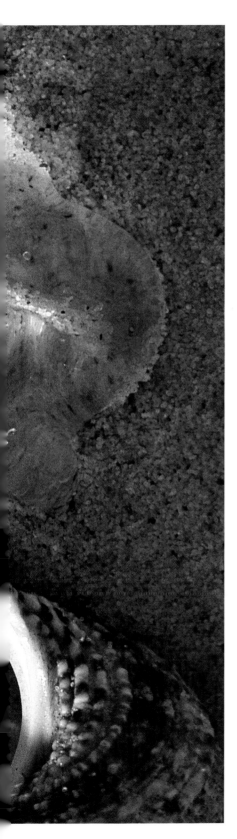

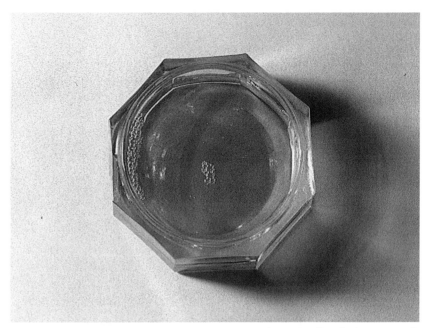

Avocado oil and wheatgerm oil.

Body lotion

3 1/2 tbsp almond or jojoba oil
2 tbsp granulated lecithin
3 1/2 tbsp glycerol
7 tbsp distilled water or orange-blossom water
1 pinch sodium benzoate if desired
4 tbsp aloe jelly

Dissolve the granulated lecithin in the oil, using a water-bath, and allow the liquid to become really hot. Meanwhile, heat the water or orange-blossom water in a saucepan. If sodium benzoate is to be used, dissolve it in the liquid and not in the oil. When the granulated lecithin has dissolved, add the glycerol while stirring all the time. Remove the dish from the water-bath and add the liquid slowly, whisking constantly with an electric whisk. After a little while, add the aloe jelly and continue whisking until the lotion has cooled down completely. Keep the lotion in a dark-coloured bottle, in a cool, dark place.

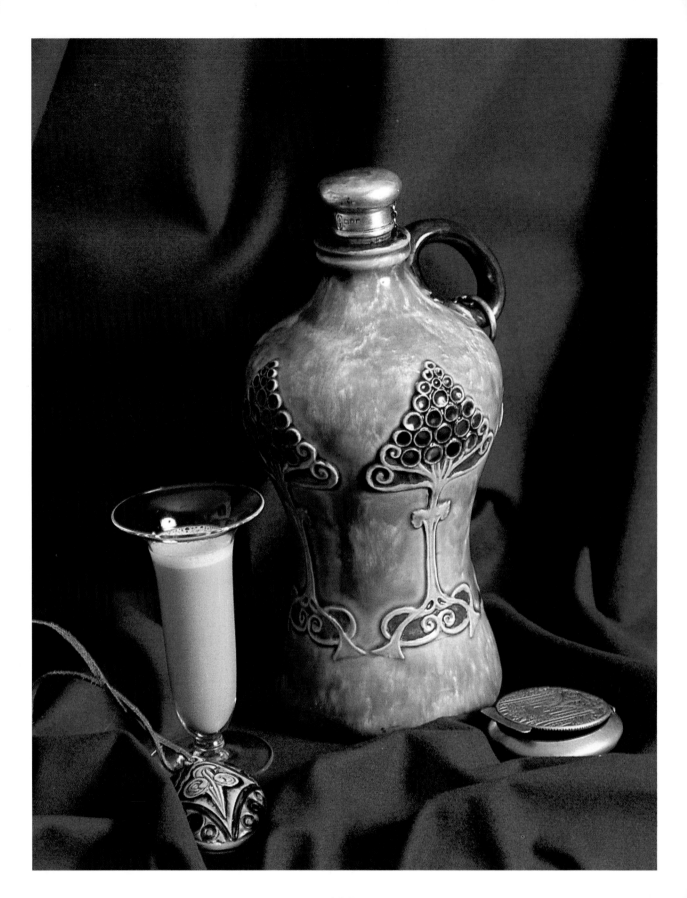

ACKNOWLEDGMENTS

The author and photographer would like to thank the following for their kind assistance in preparing this book.

Anne-Louise Barbosa
Karl-Henrik Bengtsson
Louise Berglund
The Botanical Gardens, Gothenburg
Anita Ekestubbe
Kristina Jendle
Richard Lachenardière
Helen Larsson
Eva Lindberg
Museum of Medical History, Gothenburg
Sigvor Nyström, Marabou Ltd.
Tony Reuter
Ann Louise Rönsberg
Anne Bell Watkins

Peach lotion.

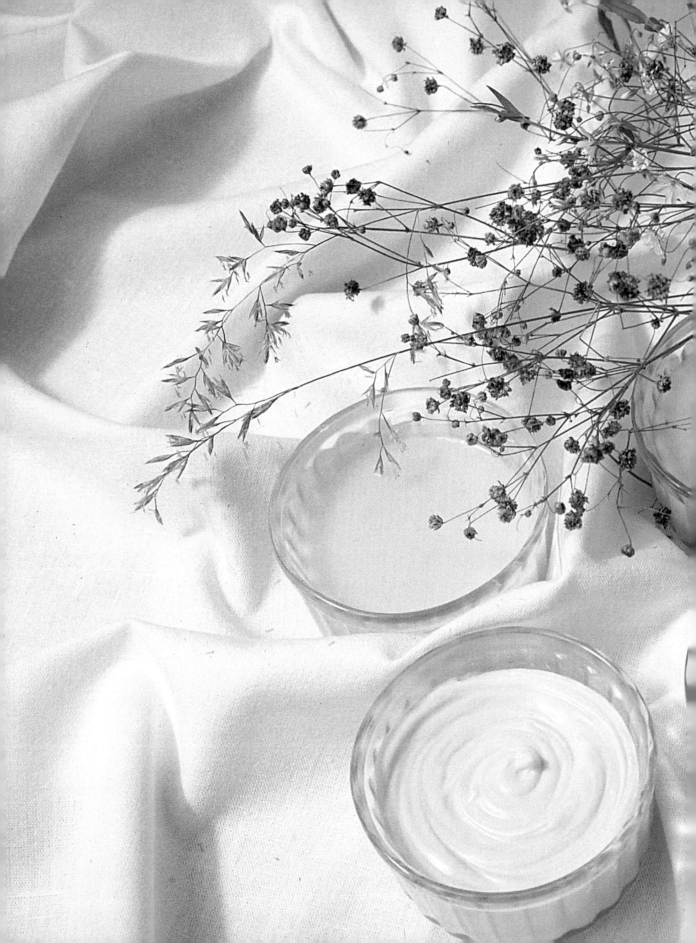

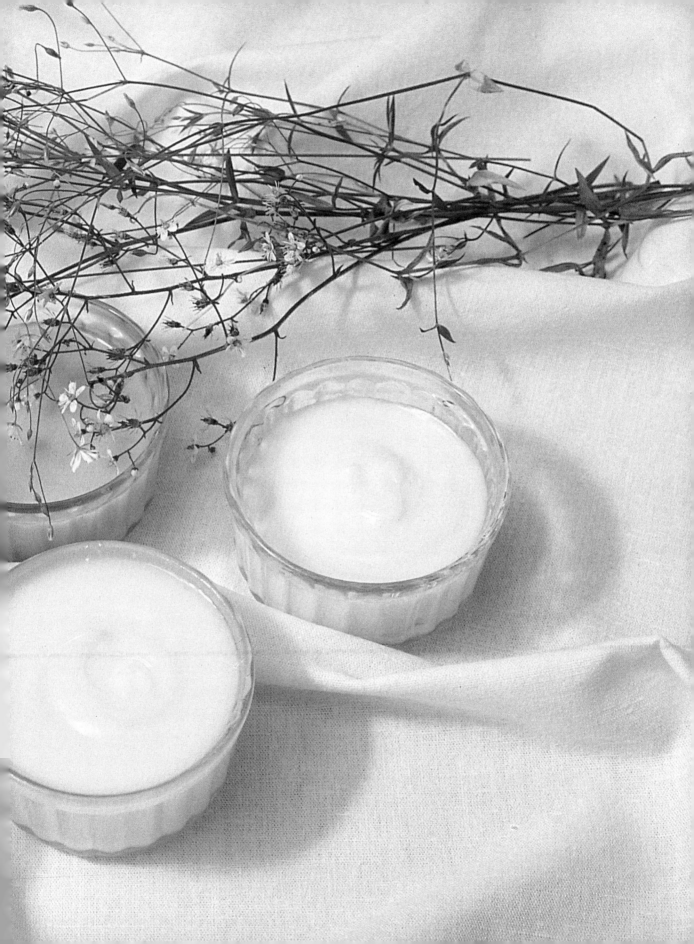

INDEX